S0-ANO-330

HEALTHY ENERGY

A good diet is essential to healthful conditioning and maximum performance in every activity. Dr. Creff's eight-year nutritional study of 15,000 athletes, including his intensive work with Olympic competitors, has yielded a simple-to-maintain diet plan that works naturally to provide maximum energy efficiency for any physical endeavor from acrobatics to zen archery.

For quick reference, Dr. Creff groups our common foods into his diet's categories, comments on the side effects certain foods can produce, and warns against some foods that athletes should never eat. He also covers essential minerals and vitamins, cholesterol, calories and liquids, as well as "protein-stuffing" and other "tricks."

Written in a clear and informative style, this book is valuable to people at all levels of athletic competence. It's a diet that works—and *the* diet that will work for you!

MORE FANTASTIC READING FROM ZEBRA!

GONJI #1: DEATHWIND OF VEDUN   (1006, $3.25)
by T. C. Rypel
Cast out from his Japanese homeland, Gonji journeys across
barbaric Europe in quest of Vedun, the distant city in the loftiest
peaks of the Alps. Brandishing his swords with fury and skill, he is
determined to conquer his hardships and fulfill his destiny!

GONJI #2: SAMURAI STEEL   (1072, $3.25)
by T. C. Rypel
His journey to Vedun is ended, but Gonji's most treacherous
battle ever is about to begin. The invincible King Klann has
occupied Vedun with his hordes of murderous soldiers—and
plotted the samurai's destruction!

CHRYSALIS 9   (1077, $2.50)
Edited by Roy Torgeson
From astronauts and time travelers, to centaurs and telepaths,
these tales of the inexplicable and the bizarre promise to astound
you!

SURVIVORS   (1071, $3.25)
by John Nahmlos
It would take more than courage and skill, more than ammo and
guns, for Colonel Jack Dawson to survive the advancing nuclear
war. It was the ultimate test—protecting his loved ones, defending
his country, and rebuilding a civilization out of the ashes of war-
ravaged America!

THE SWORD OF HACHIMAN   (1104, $3.50)
by Lynn Guest
Destiny returned the powerful sword of Hachiman to mighty
Samurai warrior Yoshitsune so he could avenge his father's brutal
death. Only he was unaware his most perilous enemy would be his
own flesh and blood!

*Available wherever paperbacks are sold, or order direct from the
Publisher. Send cover price plus 50¢ per copy for mailing and
handling to Zebra Books, 475 Park Avenue South, New York,
N.Y. 10016. DO NOT SEND CASH.*

THE MAXIMUM PERFORMANCE SPORTS DIET

BY DR. ALBERT CREFF
AND ROBERT WERNICK

(Published in hardcover as Dr. Creff's 1-2-3 Sports Diet)

ZEBRA BOOKS
KENSINGTON PUBLISHING CORP.

ZEBRA BOOKS

are published by

KENSINGTON PUBLISHING CORP.
475 Park Avenue South
New York, N.Y. 10016

Copyright © 1979 by Albert Francois Creff and Robert
Wernick. Originally published as DR. CREFF'S 1-2-3
SPORTS DIET. Reprinted by arrangement with Coward,
McCann & Geoghegan, a division of Putnam Publishing
Group.

All rights reserved. No part of this book may be reproduced
in any form or by any means without the prior written con-
sent of the Publisher, excepting brief quotes used in reviews.

Printed in the United States of America

To
Jeanne and Marion and Ruth

CONTENTS

Foreword

Albert Creff was one of the first doctors in France to direct public attention to the issue of proper nutrition for athletes—at a time when most of us thought that a basic diet of steak, with French-fried potatoes, a hunk of cheese and a glass of hearty red wine was all we needed.

The free clinic which he founded at the Hopital Saint-Michel in Paris, open to anyone interested in sports, has seen—and still sees—the most famous athletes pass through its doors. It was there that I met the great cyclist Louison Bobet, three-time winner of the Tour de France, which is probably the most severe test of physical endurance in the world of sports—its events include circling France in less than twenty-one days, 3,000 miles of straining over high mountain passes, racing at thirty miles an hour through the torrid heat of the south, battling gales on the Atlantic coast. There I also ran into Jacques Anquetil, winner of the Tour five times and holder of the world's record for racing against the clock. The skiers, gymnasts, rowers, boxers, soccer and rugby players of the last twenty years have all been guided by Dr. Creff and his staff to the discovery of the complex world of nutrition, and all agree that they have profited immensely from it.

In 1962, when I came back from the war in Algeria, I was the young hope of French skiing, but I had been weakened by amebic dysentery and drastically thinned down by viral hepatitis. Dr. Creff put me back on my feet. He was continually at the side of the French ski team during its great years 1960 and 1968 when it was practically unbeatable, achieving the unique feat of winning sixteen out of twenty-four medals at Portillo, Chile, in 1966.

Dr. Creff was at the Grenoble Olympics, which crowned General de Gaulle's efforts to give back to France some of its ancient splendor in sports. I was the big favorite that year, and I did win all three gold medals in spite of terrible physical and nervous tension. There was no more concerned spectator than Dr. Creff.

For me this was the climax of fifteen years of work on the slopes. For French skiing it was the result and reward of revolutionary techniques and discipline. For Dr. Creff it was living proof of the value of his work. He too deserves a Gold Medal.

Jean-Claude Killy
France, December 1978

Introduction

Throw away your bathroom scales! The rousing injunction with which Dr. Creff opens his first chapter indicates that he is offering a very different kind of diet book.

This is a diet to make you look better and feel better. It is only secondarily interested in helping you lose weight, though you may well lose weight as a bonus when you follow it.

This may sound like heresy to the army of weight watchers that stalks our land, hunting down the tons of fat which hang around the great American middle. Every few months a new prophet appears to rally this devoted band around a new banner—low carbohydrate or high fiber, blackstrap molasses or country vinegar or fermented mare's milk—and for a brief period becomes the focal point of thousands of lives. The results are always sensational, as satisfied testimonials bear witness. Yet isn't it odd that a new product or process or gimmick has to be brought forth so often? Isn't it probable there is something inadequate about all of them? Isn't it, in fact, all too clear to anyone who walks down the street with open eyes that, the more weight-reducing diet books sold, the fatter everybody seems to get?

Dr. Creff suggests there is a good reason why all these miracle diets are indeed inadequate, why they come on so strong and are so soon forgotten. The trouble is that they abstract a single factor—your weight—without looking at the picture of your whole self. Furthermore, they set a negative goal—taking off pounds—and it is hard to keep your energies mobilized indefinitely toward a negative goal.

This book's goal is a positive one: it is physical fitness, feeling good all over and proud of your body. The first necessary step toward such a goal is to eat correctly.

How can you be sure you are eating correctly? One simple way is to model your diet on one which has proven best for people to whom physical fitness is an absolute necessity, an underpinning for their whole way of life. In modern society, the largest class of people falling into this category is the athlete, professional and amateur. Whatever food keeps him in fittest form is bound to be good for the rest of the population as well.

Such was the line of reasoning that led Albert François Creff to write this book. He was uniquely qualified to do so. He is a specialist in metabolic diseases and heads a clinic at a large Paris hospital where some 50,000 obese people have been treated. However, his main concern over the years has not been the study of morbid states, but the care and feeding of healthy non-obese young men and women who are practicing some form of sport. Dr. Creff was nutritional adviser to the French teams at six Olympic Games, and he knows the practical requirements of athletes intimately.

It was accident that led him into this field. He was a young doctor practicing in the gastro-intestinal service of a hospital in Paris when, one summer day in 1955, a patient was brought in moaning and clutching his middle. He was a professional bicycle-racer named Fernand Picot, and he had collapsed in the middle of one of the first laps of the Tour de France, the 21-day bike race around the country which provides an annual outlet for national hysteria. Picot was complaining of unendurable pains, but the standard tests indicated no identifiable organic disease. Young Dr. Creff thought it might be useful to question him about his diet: what had he been eating during the weeks he was in training for the gruelling race over asphalt roads in mid-summer? Oh, he replied, the usual hearty French fare, *boeuf bourguignon* and such—succulent dishes smothered in rich gravy, accompanied by mountains of French-fries and washed down with pitchers of red wine and a little Pernod.

Why don't you try a slightly different diet, suggested Dr. Creff. He put his patient on a bland, balanced ration of hospital food. Within a few days the pains had gone away. Within a few weeks, Fernand Picot was back in the saddle, and the following year he won several laps of the Tour de France.

This episode influenced the young physician in the direction of what was to become his overriding lifetime interest: finding the best combination of foods for optimum performance in any kind of competition.

Nutrition for athletes was a field he had to pioneer. The shelves of medical libraries were crammed with works describing the past century's advances in our knowledge of how the human body turns food into energy. But despite the increasingly important role of competitive sports in modern life, there was no overall work on athletic nutrition in print. In fact, there had been no such study since the ancient Greeks. Albert Creff determined to provide one, and, after years of research, he did. He has been compared to another French reviver of a rich and half-forgotten Hellenic tradition: the baron de Coubertin who founded the modern Olympic Games in 1896.

It was not that the subject of food for athletes had lacked for attention. Athletes everywhere have been used to eating at training tables, following special diets and fads like anyone else. Every coach and trainer has had his own special secret for pepping up his charges, has set up strict rules and responded with the wrath of God when the rules were broken. While some of these rules, diets and fads are quite sensible, others are utter nonsense and none is based on scientific observation of evidence. Many are no more than old saws and superstitions handed down from generation to generation by other trainers, other coaches, and their grandmothers.

Dr. Creff was the first to approach the problem in a spirit of scientific enquiry. He has studied more than 15,000 athletes of all levels of competence. His major work, spanning eight years, began with an intensive examination of some 400 young men and women. Some were Olympic competitors or international superstars such as Jean-Claude Killy. He then narrowed these 400 down to 100, choosing only those who seemed to be successful in their overall life as well as in their sporting discipline; they were more or less happily married, they held down jobs, they didn't go on monthly benders or commit themselves to psychiatric hospitals.

He watched these 100 relatively normal young people closely while they were in training, while they were in competition, and while they were relaxing after competition. He kept careful note of their physical shape, careful score of their performances, and at the same time he played discreetly with their daily intake of food. One month they might eat a little more protein, the next a little more fat. Some days they might be allowed an extra dessert, or an extra glass of wine. Then he could note what, if any, changes these small shifts in their diet might have had on the way they performed in the field.

Observations like these had to be handled with caution. Nutrition is not an exact science—far from it, whatever you may have heard to the contrary from the learned men who are always bombarding you with advice on what and how to eat. The classic studies of the effect of diet on physical performance have been made in places like shoe factories. They are all a little suspect because it is difficult to make sure that what is being measured is only the effect of the diet. If a man, for example, produces more shoes on a day when he is eating more protein, it is not necessarily the protein that is responsible for the improvement: it may be that the union has just signed a favorable contract, or that his mother-in-law is leaving town. In addition, it is well known in the testing fraternity that the mere act of testing someone tends to improve his performance. He might be flattered by the attention, making him feel better and in turn enabling him to work harder without getting tired. The attention is probably more important than the food: in one famous test, factory workers' performance improved dramatically when they were given more nutritionally sound meals; but then when they were deliberately given nutritionally unsound meals, their performance went on improving, presumably out of their sheer pleasure in being the object of so much interest.

Unlike factory workers, athletes are used to being watched; they live in a fishbowl. And they are used to being tested; in fact their careers consist largely of being rated and scored in a series of tests called games, matches, races or whatnot. So they make good subjects for the kind of testing Creff was interested in.

Naturally, there was always the possibility that the individual chance event might influence the results. If a skier did poorly one month when he was eating more fat than usual, the real reason might not be the fat but a spat with his girl friend. However, if many reacted the same way, and the same effect could be observed in other sports, it was logical to conclude that this particular fat ration was well above the ideal for human consumption.

11

The next month there would be less fat on the menus, and it could be seen if performance improved.

By making thousands of such careful observations, Dr. Creff could finally work out the ideal proportions of fats, proteins and carbohydrates needed in a day's meals for maximum physical efficiency. Almost every nutritionist agreed that a balanced diet was best, but here was a way to determine exactly *how* it should be balanced, to the nearest percentage point. Creff's percentages—15 for protein, 30 for fat, 55 for carbohydrate—are now generally accepted as standard by nutritionists throughout the world.

The eight years of study and research (three of them on the selected group of 100 athletes) finally led to his writing a thick volume called *Sport et Alimentation*, first published in France in 1963 and now recognized as the classic in its field. It has been translated into most European languages.

This first English-language version is a deliberately simplified one, prepared in collaboration with Dr. Creff. It is meant for the layman and not the specialist. It contains the basic matter of the original volume, brought up to date where necessary, stripped of its apparatus of charts, footnotes and summaries of articles in medical journals. We have tried to suppress technical jargon and write in plain language for the ordinary reader. Students who would like to see for themselves the technical background and statistical support for statements made here are referred to the latest French edition (La Table Ronde, Paris, 1969).

The specific purpose of this book is to make you feel better, look better, perform better, whether you are a professional athlete aiming at a world championship, a daily jogger, a Sunday golfer or one of the legion of pajama-clad hoppers and jumpers emulating the Royal Canadian Air Force—anyone, in short, who is trying to keep in some minimum of shape. You may well lose some weight in the process, but that is not the primary consideration. We do not propose a reducing diet, but a building diet, one that will help you acquire and preserve a healthy, energetic body.

You do not have to be an Olympic competitor or a physical fitness nut to profit by it. The book is based on experience among athletes, and it is aimed at an audience of athletes. But every one of us has to be an athlete at some moments or periods of our lives. Just as the most dedicated runner or football-player cannot possibly keep in training all the time—he has to let the bars down every so often and swill down some forbidden sweets—so the rest of us, the soft and sedentary, the lazy, the deskbound, cannot drift through our whole lives in flabby inactivity and self-indulgence. There are times when we have to be up and about our business with all the concentration and devotion of a competitor in the decathlon. We may have an election to win, an examination to pass, a deal to clinch, a weekend to pass with a dream-object, and on such occasions even we have to be strong, alert, in tiptop shape, at the height of our powers. And of course there are professions, such as ballet dancing, which may make demands on the body every bit as arduous as those imposed by any sport.

So everyone can find something of value in this book. It is useless to expect this or any other book to do it all for you. To get into good shape you have to take some physical exercise; in what form and how much is entirely up to you. What the book can do is show you what and how to eat so that you can get the greatest possible advantage out of that physical exercise.

You will find that Dr. Creff is an understanding guide, and he will not ask you to do anything too difficult. There are no absolute prohibitions in his diet—"there are no forbidden fruits," as he says, "you just have to know how to bite them." The right way to bite them may involve taking somewhat fewer bites than you would like, but the range of foods available to you is as wide as the earth.

Naturally, if you take up any diet at all, you must expect to have to sacrifice something you like. Otherwise, it would hardly be a diet. Fourteen years ago, I wrote, pseudonymously, a little pamphlet called *The Drinking Man's Diet* which achieved a certain success. On three continents I have seen grateful readers make their way toward me, often on unsteady feet, to thank me effusively for having saved their lives or, as they often put it, enabled them to have their cake and eat it too. This mustn't be taken literally: cakes are frowned on in the Drinking Man's, as in most other diets. (But not, as you will see, in Dr. Creff's.) However, it is true that no other diet can compare to the Drinking Man's in allowing sheer joy to prevail in the dining room. Where else can you find one that allows you gourmet dishes plus unlimited quantities of wine, champagne (but only the best champagne) and whisky? People around the world still follow this diet, and still hiccup their thanks in my direction.

My earlier readers will perhaps think I am turning traitor by presenting this book, with a diet which is admittedly more Spartan and on the whole hostile to the consumption of alcohol.

But I am not abandoning any principles. I still maintain that the Drinking Man's Diet—as so many other diets on the market—is perfectly valid for a specific purpose. In this case, the purpose is to enable you to drink your fill and eat enough to satisfy your hunger, without getting grossly fat in the process. There may be periods in your life—say you are a traveling salesman duty-bound to match your customers glass for glass over many consecutive meals—when such a regimen is absolutely essential.

However, looking at your life as a whole, there is no guarantee all that wine, champagne and whisky is going to be good for you. If you are going in seriously for athlet-

14

ics or any other activity demanding top fitness, it is apt to be bad for you. And even from a purely hedonistic point of view, the Drinking Man's Diet is not without certain inconveniences. Its anti-carbohydrate bias entails cutting out virtually all fruits and vegetables, and when following it I have often been overcome with frustrated desire for crisp green garden peas or a ripe juicy peach.

The present volume has a much broader outlook and goal. It is aimed at making you, the whole you, function better throughout your life.

Dr. Creff is wordly-wise enough to know that you will not follow his advice all of the time, and rarely will you follow it to the letter. However, if you follow only the general outlines of his diet, you will be doing yourself a great deal of good. Even if you don't, you will find valuable hints and information scattered through these chapters that may at least help keep you out of trouble.

You will not have to revolutionize your diet to follow him. He touts no miracle product, he brings you none of the aerobic kit and macrobiotic caboodle with which the seers and shamans of the nutritionistic world offer to remake you. Common sense is his watchword, and he wants you to go on eating the common foods you are used to, though you may be taking more of some and less of others.

His approach is pragmatic throughout. What has helped all the athletes he has worked with? What specifically will help you?

He starts in Chapter I with a few simple principles. He tells you why to diet and how to go about it.

In Chapter II, he shows you how to apply these principles in a form so simple that you can follow it anywhere, at home or away from home, without taking more than a moment's thought. No need to pull out a chart and start counting laboriously every time you sit down to eat. Unlike so many other diets which call for feats of mathematical computation, this one demands no intellectual effort greater than counting to four. You will have a handy practical guide to daily eating that can help you, all at once, get rid of bad habits which have piled up over a lifetime.

Chapter III tells you, in simple non-technical language, all you have to know about the science of nutrition in order to understand the reasons behind the advice you are being given.

Chapter IV gives the details of the ideal diet worked out by Dr. Creff on his athletes, one that you can use as a model for the rest of your life.

Chapter V contains an alphabetical listing of most of the common foods you eat, rated according to their value for physical fitness, and accompanied by lively comments based on a lifetime of medical experience. Here is a chance for you to learn, for example, why it is advisable to peel your tomatoes (p. 143) or why women should go easy on premium beer (p. 112).

Chapter VI gives an alphabetical list of sports, from archery to weight lifting, via backgammon, Ping-Pong and spelunking. It gives practical advice about what, when and how to eat while you are practicing them.

In Chapter VII he turns to a vital question which has been almost entirely neglected by other authorities: what do you eat in the day or so *after* intense physical effort, when your body is feeling its way back to normal?

Chapter VIII takes a brief look at a subject which is of perennial interest in many countries besides the Doctor's native France, to wit, the relation between diet and sex.

And the last chapter takes up some of the troubles athletes or others can get into through improper eating habits, and the often surprisingly simple ways of getting out of them.

In short, you have here a wide and rich repertory of useful knowledge. It is not the answer to all your bodily problems, but it is a good beginning, and that is what you

16

need. As the lady said when asked if she believed that Saint Dionysius could really have walked the three miles from Montmartre to St. Denis with his freshly cut-off head in his hands, *c'est le premier pas qui compte:* the first step is the big one.

ROBERT WERNICK

APPROXIMATE METRIC EQUIVALENTS

Weight

1 gram (g)	.035	ounces (oz)
1 kilogram (kg)	2.205	pounds (lb)
1 ounce	28.5	grams
1 pound	.453	kilograms

Volume

1 milliliter (mL)	.03	fluid ounces (fl oz)
1 liter (L)	1.06	quarts (qt)
1 tablespoon (Tbsp)	15	milliliters
1 fluid ounce	30	milliliters
1 cup (c)	.24	liters
1 quart	.95	liters

I
Beginning to Diet

The best way to begin to diet is to throw away your bathroom scales.

They are probably inaccurate to begin with, and more importantly, they start your day's thinking off in the wrong direction. It is easy to become fascinated by those tiny lines and figures and translate them into vexatious emotional states. There are women I know who groan and moan if the needle passes 125 pounds; at 130 they start having nightmares; at 135 they talk of suicide. This is silly at best, and totally wrong-headed. For remember that what you see on the scales are figures, that is to say abstractions. When you say, "I have a pimple on my nose," or "I feel fine today," you are dealing with something concrete and verifiable. But 125 pounds by itself is only a figure in the void. It has to be interpreted in the light of your entire physical and mental structure.

Pounds are abstract, therefore pounds are neutral. A pound of muscle weighs the same as a pound of fat. A

21

pound of well-distributed flesh that makes you feel pleasantly relaxed weighs as much as a pound that hangs like a dead weight around your stomach.

So the first step toward rational dieting is this: stop thinking of yourself as an arithmetical figure and concentrate on your tangible, visible figure instead. Replace the scales by a full-length mirror; take off all your clothes and take an honest look at yourself. If you are pleased with what you see, what are you worrying about? You may find many helpful hints in a book like this which will improve your overall fitness, but you should think very carefully about rushing into any sudden change of diet. Why monkey with any part of a way of life which has brought about such a splendid sight as now appears in your mirror?

On the other hand, suppose the mirror offers you an unpleasant collection of bumps and bulges. You will naturally want to get rid of them even if the chart says that your weight is correct for your height and build.

I have often seen patients insist they were not overweight because a chart told them so, when a pinch at their midriff could prove the opposite. And conversely, I have seen many athletes, superb collections of muscle and sinew, literally starve themselves to get down to a weight their charts told them was ideal, eating up some of their precious muscle in the process and throwing their whole system out of kilter. Unless you are bound by the strict rules of some sport like boxing or horse-racing, it is pointless to pay much attention to weight charts. What you want is the weight that fits you, personally, best, that goes with your looking good and feeling healthy. When you have found that weight, you should try to stick to it. But it is a waste of time and nervous energy to be testing it on the scales every day, to see if it has fluctuated a few ounces. Mother Nature does not think in pounds and ounces, and you needn't either.

Now, let us suppose that you have made the mirror test and, as so many of your compatriots, you are not at all pleased: this, surely, is not what you intend to stuff into a bikini and expose to the eyes of all the people on the beach.

If it is only a matter of a few bulges (and if summer is still a good way off), there is no reason to be concerned. A few weeks of exercise and a rational balanced diet will get you into acceptable shape. But if you are uncomfortably overweight, if you find yourself really unsightly in your mirror, you will want to start your diet by taking off some pounds quickly.

This may sound a little strange. Isn't the whole *aim* of dieting, you may ask, to take off pounds quickly?

Not at all. The aim of dieting is to keep you alive and alert and healthy. You are going to start your serious dieting *after* you have taken off those unnecessary pounds.

Despite what you have been told all your life, and perhaps firmly believed on the basis of your own experience, it is not at all difficult to lose weight. All you have to do—unless you are suffering from glandular or psychological disturbances which are outside the scope of this book—is to eat less.

I understand that an American doctor has pushed this principle to its logical extreme, and made a good deal of money in the process, by recommending what he calls the ultimate diet, which means going without any food at all—for limited periods, I assume. This is the oldest and most tried of reducing systems; it has kept poor people underweight since the beginning of human history.

Starvation will certainly take the pounds off, but I myself prefer a somewhat less drastic method. When athletes come to me for advice as they start their training, and I find them manifestly overweight, I put them on the following diet:

All the lean beef, veal, liver you want, provided it is grilled, roasted or boiled and served without gravy or sauce

All the poultry you want, grilled or roasted, without the skin

All the fish you want, grilled or boiled

All the green vegetables you want—fresh or cooked in boiling salted water

All the lettuce or other salad vegetable you want, with lemon juice or vinegar as dressing

All the skimmed milk you want

These foods should be taken any time you are hungry, and you should go on eating till your appetite is satisfied. If you still feel pangs of hunger between meals, you were probably suffering from malnutrition to begin with. (The fact that you were fat doesn't mean that you were well fed; quite the contrary in most cases.) Nibble at some cold cuts or take a drink of skimmed milk to repress this feeling of hunger.

The foregoing comprises your basic ration, and I repeat you can take all you want of it. The following supplements, however, should be strictly limited; do not take any more than I recommend here on any single day:

3 to 8 pieces of toast with 1 tablespoon of butter

1 tablespoon of vegetable oil (with your vegetables or salad)

1 apple

1 citrus fruit

3 to 8 lumps of sugar

1 yogurt

25 grams (about an ounce) of cheese

Plus the following, to be taken not on a daily basis but in the course of a week:

3 boiled eggs
About a dozen and a half oysters

Use as little salt as you can stand at all meals. This is
certainly no starvation diet, and will enable you to em-
bark on a program of physical effort with no difficulty or
inconvenience, except that it may be mildly constipating.
It is a deliberately unbalanced diet, which explains both
why it works and why you must not follow it too long:
give it up as soon as the proper number of pounds have
dropped off.

People to whom I propose this diet are generally in-
credulous at the outset. How can I possibly lose weight,
they cry, with no restrictions on the amount of meat and
all those other things I can eat? The answer is perfectly
simple.

In the first place, the most important factor in a weight-
reducing program is *not to be hungry.* If you are hungry,
not only is your efficiency lowered and your whole life
disorganized, but your body is constantly urging you to
cheat. And sooner or later you will cheat, undoing all the
good work when you started out with such good inten-
tions.

The diet I propose is extremely high in proteins and
protein-rich food is eminently satisfying to the appetite.
Your body uses as much protein as it needs for building
up and repairing its own structure, and eliminates the
rest; it cannot stock any, to add pounds to your weight.

The diet is also rich in cellulose (in the green vegetables), which has no nutritive value but adds bulk, to keep
your digestion going smoothly.

It is very low in fat and carbohydrate, much too low for
a permanent ration. It gives you an essential minimum of
both, which will be burned up as energy and not stocked
away as fat in your body.

You must not drink any alcohol while following this

reducing diet. Your body, as if aware that this is a toxic material which should be gotten rid of immediately, burns alcohol for energy before it burns anything else. So if you drink while you eat, the alcohol will go into energy, and the food will go into deposits of fat draped unesthetically around your middle or elsewhere.

If you follow this diet, you will lose at least two pounds a week. After the appropriate number of weeks, stop. A high-protein diet under normal circumstances is both useless (since your body gets rid of the protein it does not need) and expensive (as you learn every day at the butcher shop); and it can put a strain on your liver and kidneys.

Perhaps you will not share my enthusiasm for this weight-reducing diet. Perhaps you are devoted to some other system, or have heard of a new miracle method which can slim you down in no time with no trouble. There are, I am informed, some 217 reducing diets currently on the market in the Western world, not to speak of the hundreds more which are out of print but which can be found tucked away in old bookcases and second-hand bookstores. None of them, so far as I know, is specifically poisonous. It is true that many of them can upset your system badly and be dangerous to your health if you follow them for long periods, but it is very unlikely that you will adhere to any of them very long. Therefore, for the limited purpose of losing weight in a hurry, I will not object too strongly if you choose any one of these 217 rivals that strikes your fancy.

The reason I don't object is that experience has taught me that all diets work—for a while. They work because they all, in one way or another, demand cutting down on the food you used to eat, and if you eat less food you will sooner or later lose weight.

This pleasing result, however, will last only as long as you are able to follow your diet exactly, precisely, every day, week after week. And if you are an average human being, you simply won't be able to do that. Either you will lose interest, or your body, your long-suffering body, will rise up and rebel and force you to abandon the unwelcome, painful (and often dangerous) disciplines you are imposing on it.

It is true that the human body is an almost infinitely adjustable organism, and people have been known to live and apparently to flourish on the oddest of diets, which any nutritionist would call hopelessly inadequate. There are people in Melanesia who live on a diet consisting largely of yams, there are Eskimos in the frozen north who spend months eating nothing but walrus blubber. But they eat what they do because they have no other choice. You do have a choice, and it is folly to try to follow their example. Man is an omniverous animal, and his nutrition should ideally cover the whole spectrum of edible foods. If you deprive yourself of any of them, you are at best giving your body a problem of adjustment and at worst depriving yourself of something necessary and laying yourself open to disease. In my clinical work I have often seen women who have been hysterically trying to follow a sensational new crash diet they saw in the glossy pages of a magazine and who are literally starving, their bodies wasting away, like the Biafrans in the war a few years back.

It need not come to that. Generally your body comes to your rescue, it lets you know it is missing the good old foods it craves, it encourages you to cheat. As the initial burst of enthusiasm wears off, you find yourself breaking the rules, more or less absent-mindedly, on more and more occasions. You scoop up a handful of nuts at a cocktail party, and forget to add it to your record of the day's intake. Pretty soon you forget to count the cocktails too. You are invited out, and offered tempting dishes, and you decide that just this once you will make an exception. As the days go by, there are more exceptions than rules.

In addition, most diets are bores. They demand complicated forms of counting, and I suspect that there is something built into our genetic structure which recoils from dealing with numbers larger than our 20 fingers and toes. It may be fun for the first few days to total up quantities of calories or grams of carbohydrates but after a while it gets to be a burden to pull out the charts and tote up all the figures.

This is just about the time to forget your miracle diet. It will have performed its only function, which is to get your weight down. Once it is down to a reasonable figure, stop worrying about it. What I am going to propose now is a course of action designed to get you into good shape. If you follow it, your weight problems will be solved more or less automatically.

Half of the program is up to you, and is outside the scope of this book. I assume that you are performing or preparing to perform some regular and rather vigorous physical exercise. Without it, no amount of sensible nutrition is going to give you a body beautiful to admire in that mirror.

My diet is for people with healthy appetites. You don't need to be a full-time athlete to have that, but neither can you expect to develop one by sitting in an easy-chair all day watching television. The modern work-week is short enough, and facilities for exercise are universal enough, so that there is little excuse for not getting in sufficient physical activity every week to keep you in good shape.

I also assume that you have sense enough to see a doctor before you start tinkering with your eating habits. I have too often seen tragic results when people who have not had a physical examination for years rush abruptly into radical diets which can hurt or even kill them.

The advice I will be giving in this book is for the average healthy man and woman. The chances are very strong that that is just what you are, but there are plenty of exceptional cases walking the streets, and you owe it to yourself to find out if you are one of them. There are many common diseases such as diabetes which demand a spe-

28

cial diet, and only a qualified physician can tell you what it is. And there are all sorts of uncommon conditions too.

If you read medical texts, you will discover dozens of diseases and syndromes which result in obesity. You may have suffered damage to your hypothalamus gland, disturbing the body's mechanism of warning you, through hunger, when you need to eat; so you eat irrationally, unnecessarily. Various hormones may get off the track as they are apt to do at moments of bodily change such as puberty or menopause. Psychological disturbances notoriously can drive people to overeating and putting on fat. There are (happily rare) diseases such as the Klein-Lewin Syndrome, whose unhappy victims sleep 22 hours a day and can think only of eating and making love in the remaining two.

If you read the whole list, you may wonder why everyone on earth isn't hopelessly fat. But the fact is that such disorders affect only a small minority of mankind. Most of us, at least in our prosperous hygienic modern world, are in relatively satisfactory good health, and there is nothing to prevent us trying to make it better by some comparatively small improvements in our diet.

It is important to emphasize at the outset that your diet is not an isolated phenomenon which you can consider independently, apart from the rest of your life. Man does not live by food alone. This is often overlooked by nutritionists, whose professional vice is to think of the body as merely a digestive machine which needs only to be fed the proper nutrients in the proper quantities in order to function at peak efficiency. Unfortunately for them (but fortunately for us) the real world is more complicated than that. There is an authoritarian streak in many experts, well captured in the scene in *Modern Times* where the learned professor straps Charlie Chaplin down so that he can be fed properly. I sometimes get the impression that nutritionists would be happier if we were all fed out of troughs of identical food which would run past our work-benches at stated hours of the day, and we would all ingest identical portions at the same time and all remain as a result in identical states of good health. The world has not quite come to that, and I don't anticipate that it ever will.

Every one of us is an individual, with our own individual tastes, preferences, prejudices, quirks, and no diet that doesn't allow you to express them can succeed in the long run. As you will see when I spell out specific recommendations for daily meals, there is no single item of food which you absolutely must eat—there is always a substitute available. And equally true, there is no item which you absolutely must *not* eat. There are no forbidden fruits—you only have to know how to bite them. There must be room for individual liberty, here as in other spheres of life.

Another great temptation for nutritionists is to isolate a single phenomenon in the digestive process, build a theory on it, and then try to force the whole world to revolutionize its eating habits on the basis of the theory. It has been seriously argued, for example, by men with medical degrees and other credentials, that because the human gut is quite long, like that of fruit-eating monkeys, human beings are therefore biologically fruit-eaters, and if we want to be really healthy we should give up everything else. (Proponents of this theory have a wonderful time describing the noisome stinking mass into which meat turns in the intestines, as opposed to the pleasantly bland one formed by fruit.) I am not enough of a paleoanthropologist to say if the length of our intestines is a relic of fruit-eating days in an Eocenic past. But I do have enough practical experience to assure you that, if you follow the advice of these experts and stick to an exclusive diet of bananas, you will not only be bored to death, you will get a perpetual stomachache, and you won't help yourself win medals in tree-climbing or any other sport.

This is a good example of focusing on one detail (in

this case the length of the intestines) and using it arbitrarily to change the whole dietary picture. It is easy to play this game, and the results are almost always absurd. There is a useful measurement known to nutritionists as the coefficient of net protein use. Its basic function is to measure the ease with which proteins in your food can be transformed into the proteins which build up your own body cells. The lower the coefficient, the less time and energy your body has to spend on the work of transformation; and therefore, the less food you have to eat.

This is clearly advantageous, as well as economical. But if you tried to build your whole diet around this single factor, you would soon get into trouble. The food with the lowest coefficient, hence the one most efficiently absorbed by the human organism, is human flesh. It has been shown that frogs do best on frog meat, and dogs on dog meat, but current prejudices being what they are, I doubt if we will ever see a scientific test of cannibals versus beef-eaters in any athletic pursuit. Next lowest coefficient after human flesh belongs to eggs, but eggs are unfortunately high in cholesterol, and you should not eat them every day. After eggs comes dog meat, which was a delicacy among the ancient Aztecs (and still is in some provinces of China, where they breed fat yellow puppies for the purpose) but you would get an unfavorable reaction if you fed it to your guests today. And after dog meat comes pig meat, which ordinarily has too high a fat content to be recommended for a steady diet.

In short, while it is a good thing to know that there is a coefficient of protein use, we would have to take a great many other things—social and psychological as well as physical—into account before we could begin using it to make up rules of nutrition.

Our present state of nutritional knowledge does not permit us to make iron-clad rules at all. I believe the only practical way to proceed is empirically. Let us examine the best and fittest specimens, men and women who by the very nature of what they do have to be in good condition, the very best condition. Athletes are an obvious choice. If we can determine the forms and styles of nourishment that keep them in the best possible shape, then these forms and styles should be good for the average man and woman too.

This was the principle followed by the ancient Greeks, who may be said to have invented both athletics and the study of nutrition. From the earliest times the Greeks set great store by games, and the leading runners and wrestlers and so on were regarded as heroic figures, their feats recorded in poem and statuary. It was natural for the doctors who were beginning the scientific study of the human body to give particular attention to the feeding of athletes.

There were two schools among these doctors. One, associated with names such as Dromeus of Stymphalus, recommended different diets for different forms of physical exertion. Let the racer eat antelope meat, they said, the jumper eat goat meat, the wrestler bull meat. The origins of these ideas may go back to primitive magical lore, as when the cannibal eats the heart of a brave enemy to increase his own strength and courage. But Dromeus and his supporters presented them as scientific fact. And there are successors of Dromeus who are still so presenting them today.

There are reputable nutritionists, for example, who maintain that sports demanding brief exertion, such as sprints, call for a completely different diet from those which require long endurance, such as the marathon. They recommend a high-protein diet for the former and a high-carbohydrate diet for the latter, pointing to the way runners from countries where the staple diet is rice, manioc and other cereals, have won so many championships in distance runs.

I do not agree at all. For one thing, those long-distance runners turn out on examination to have a much broader diet than rice and manioc. For another, under modern conditions competitors in all events go through much the same intensive training, and need the same reserves of energy. And on theoretical grounds, I cannot understand why carbohydrates, which are valuable for providing quick bursts of energy, should not be emphasized for sprints, and fats and proteins, which take longer to turn into energy, for long-distance events.

In my judgment it is wrong to overemphasize any one of these three components of our diet and force-feed athletes with it in the hope of giving them a temporary surplus of energy. My experience with thousands of athletes in all kinds of events and conditions leads me to side with the rival school in Greece, the one led by the great Hippocrates, father of medicine. He held that the basic diet for all forms of athletics, as for a healthy life in general, is the same. Hippocrates recommended a balanced diet with room in it for all the ordinary foods that omniverous man likes and is used to: meat, milk, vegetables, fruit, and bread, sweet and sour, fat and lean, all the wide range of edible things that God put upon the earth for our nourishment.

The soundness of Hippocrates' advice was confirmed in spectacular fashion in the later years of the Roman Empire, when in the last desperate days the state pressed into army service the gladiators who had been accustomed to perform in the Coliseum at Rome and in other cities. These men had been carefully nurtured in accordance with the principles of Dromeus; they had been given a high-protein diet consisting almost entirely of red meat. It turned them beefy enough; they made impressive figures as they swaggered around the arena chopping one another's limbs off. But when they were faced with the very different rigors of a military campaign, bivouacking and fighting barbarians in damp forests and snowy mountains, they quickly went to pieces, and their general utility to the army was nil. They would have been better soldiers—and they undoubtedly would have been better gladiators too—with a more frugal and more varied diet.

So let us mark down once and for all Hippocrates' basic principle: variety and balance are the twin pillars of a healthy diet.

There is an important proviso, however, one that Hippocrates himself was the first to insist on. No matter how clearly advantageous a balanced diet may appear, no matter how we can show that it improves performance in case after case, we must always avoid sudden or radical changes in diet when the person involved is doing all right as it is. Here again we have the principle of looking at the whole human being rather than the specific part.

I believe, for example, that it has been amply demonstrated that radical vegetarianism (that is, refusing to eat any meat or fish or animal products like eggs and milk) is nonsense and dangerous nonsense, that athletes who eat a proper combination of meat and vegetable products will do better than those who live on vegetables alone. I will preach this to vegetarians, but I will not try to force them to change their ways.

A young girl named Claude Mandonnaud once came to me for advice. She had won a few local swimming championships and wanted to go further. I found that she never touched animal protein because someone had told her it was bad for her. She had a perfectly normal body, and I recommended adding very small quantities of meat to her diet. When she discovered that they weren't poisoning her, she went on to eat more, and perhaps coincidentally, won several national and European medals.

There was no trouble here, because vegetarianism was nothing more than a teen-age fad with Claude. If it had been a firmly held religious belief, I would not have tried to meddle with it, and would have tried to find some way of readjusting her diet to give her a more or less adequate substitute for the animal protein she was giving up. The psychological effect of breaking cherished rules and risk-

34

ing all the pangs of conscience that would have ensued far outweighed any physical gain to be derived from eating meat.

Similarly, it has been repeatedly shown that Moslem athletes who practice their religion devoutly perform somewhat poorly during the month of Ramadan when they are forbidden to take any nourishment between sun-up and sundown. Obviously they would be in better shape if they kept up their regular eating hours during the Ramadan; but this would be a sacrilege, and anyone foolish enough to talk them into doing it would probably see their performances sink away to zero.

Many famous athletes have made it almost a point of honor to disregard the advice of the authorities and eat foods that are generally frowned on. Babe Ruth stayed at the top of the baseball world for nearly two decades while going through mountains of bratwurst and oceans of beer. This was very much part of his life-style, and I doubt that he would have done any better by drinking milk.

The magazine *Sports Illustrated* recently published a report on the dietary peculiarities of many leading sports figures. My eye was caught by the football player Fred Dryer who eats 70 raw eggs a week. ("Forget about cholesterol," he says—very rashly, I think.) Joe Ehrmann of the Baltimore Colts specializes in peanut butter, which he puts on toast and celery when he isn't mixing it with mayonnaise; he also dotes on beets.

Other athletes who appear in the article include vegetarians of all stripes, "megavitamin gulpers, high-carbohydrate dieters, glycogen loaders and even some who think stoking up on bee pollen will improve their performance." (Glycogen-loading is a currently fashionable revival of ancient fallacies: it calls for a diet crushingly weighted in favor of protein for three days, followed by a heavy workout which is supposed to drain the muscles of all the glycogen which supplies their energy. This is followed by a three-day high-carbohydrate session which is supposed to load the muscles with fresh glycogen, which in turn is supposed to give an added zing to performance when the big game arrives. As we will see later, there is no reason for believing it does any such thing.) Some of these athletes are extremely articulate about their preferences and can reel off paragraphs of plausible-sounding nutritional theory to support them.

So long as they are holding down their demanding jobs and satisfying their bosses or coaches and the crowds in the stadium, I see no reason for quarreling with them. Maybe they have peculiar constitutions for which these odd diets are ideally suited. I do think that Messrs. Dryer and Ehrmann are laying it on a bit thick, and I wonder if they wouldn't be still better performers if they added a little common sense to their theories. Maybe Mr. Dryer could try replacing a few of his eggs with peanut-butter sandwiches, providing a little vegetable fat and carbohydrate to weigh against all the protein and animal fat he is eating now. It has been my experience that, other things being equal, the athlete following a sound, well-balanced diet will do better than one who does not. But I would have to leave that to Mr. Dryer's judgment.

The most interesting thing, to me, in the *Sports Illustrated* article was not that athletes such as these had bizarre food preferences; it was, rather, that there were so few of them. I am informed by an editor of the magazine that queries had been sent out to correspondents all over the country asking for unusual dietary preferences on the part of local athletes. There were very few usable replies for the simple reason that most athletes tend to eat simple, well-balanced meals. They do this by a kind of autoregulation, because those are the kinds of meals they like.

I suspect that that is one of the reasons they are athletes in the first place. Just as they are stronger and better coordinated than the rest of us, so their bodies are wiser (wiser too than many coaches and trainers and nutritionists), and if they are left to their own devices they tend instinctively toward a correct combination of foods.

In *Nutrition and the Athlete,* which includes replies to a questionnaire sent out to a large number of Olympic athletes, Rod Milburn, 110-meter high hurdle champion, says, "I eat no special foods." Dave Wottle, the 800-meter record-holder: "I don't take anything artificial except Rolaids." Jim Ryun, the great miler: "I eat no special foods and take no supplements." Jeff Galloway, the 10-mile champion: "I am a firm believer in three balanced meals a day." Steve Genter, the swimmer: "I try to eat a balanced diet each day." Mark Spitz: "I don't take any supplements." Chris Taylor, of the U.S. wrestling team: "I don't believe in supplements, just a lot of regular food."

The authors of the nutrition book are appalled by such insouciance. "It seems incredible," they wail, "that many athletes who are looked up to as the paragons of physical health and culture take so little interest in diet and nutrition." They compare them to a racing-car driver who would pay no attention to the "oils, tires and engine components his car needs for maximum functioning."

I, on the other hand, say, good for Jim Ryun, Mark Spitz and the rest. I think they are taking excellent care of their oils, tires and engine components. It is possible that I might be able to suggest minor improvements in the way they balance their meals, but I should say that they are doing very well as it is, and that they should go on disregarding meddlesome nutritionists and following their own instincts.

Of course education and national prejudices can distort these instincts somewhat. American athletes are brought up in homes where there is too much fat in the daily diet. French athletes are brought up on the detestable practice of doing virtually without breakfast. But the instincts are still there.

I have had occasion to work closely with hundreds of

French athletes on the Olympic teams, and I have been able to observe hundreds more from all over the world at the Olympic Games themselves. They represent every possible approach to food: some eat like horses and some like birds; some love meat and some won't touch it; some adore and some despise sweets, seafood, sassafras tea, anything you can name. But when I have analyzed their meals over a period of time—not the meals they were fed at training tables but the meals they freely ordered when they were on their own—I have been struck again and again by the way their own tastes tend to choose a combination of protein, fat and carbohydrate in proportions which hover within a few percentage points of the ideal proportions I worked out in my eight years of concentrated research.

I will take up these proportions in a later chapter and show you in some detail both why they are important to your health and how you can translate them with a minimum of fuss into your daily diet.

But before introducing any fine details or complexities, I would like to propose to you a good preliminary diet which will give you a rough-and-ready way of achieving the ideal proportions at once, and at the same time will get you used to the all-important idea of thinking of your food in terms of proportions.

Unlike other diets which demand that you calculate in scores and hundreds of grams and calories, this one does not require you to count any higher than four.

II
It's as Simple as . . .

After I had worked out the ideal proportions for a correctly balanced diet, my assistants and I set to work making up menus which would put these proportions in practical form. Analyzing a large number of these, I found an overall pattern constantly recurring, and this led me to produce a simplified diet which can provide an approximation to the ideal ration, and thus give a boost to your general health and spirits, and at the same time will put absolutely no strain on your mental powers, no matter how tired or distracted you may be. As I have said, you won't have to count any higher than four, and if that seems too much for you, you can get by with counting to three.

Naturally this will not be an exact, scientifically calculated diet. You will pick up many other details and refinements in later chapters. But it is a good sound diet that will never get you into trouble, and if you go no further in the book than this chapter, you will have been introduced to the habit of thinking of food not as totals but as proportions, something that may prove helpful all your life. The simplicity of this diet makes it easy to slip it into the schedule of your daily life; the amount of time you will have to spend calculating what to eat will be small indeed.

It can be called the 1-2-4 (or the 1-2-3, if you don't have a sweet tooth). Or you can call it the FPC diet, after the three main components of our foods: fats, proteins, carbohydrates. It is not at all easy to know how much of each of these we actually eat, for most foods are a combination of two or all three of them. Meat is largely protein, but usually contains considerable amounts of fat. Grain products are largely carbohydrate but contain varying amounts of protein. When you get a mixed dish like an Irish stew, you need a chemist to figure out the exact proportions.

For the purposes of our 1-2-4 diet, we will disregard all these complexities. Instead of taking every food as it is, a combination of elements, we will arbitrarily put it whole in the category of its chief component.

Thus, we will count as protein and only as protein:

Meat and meat products
Fish and seafood
Eggs
Milk
Buttermilk
Cheese
Yogurt
Milk-based desserts like custard

We will count as fat and only as fat:

Butter
Cream
Margarine

Lard
Vegetable oils
Mayonnaise
Gravies and sauces
Salad dressings
Peanuts, almonds and other nuts
Peanut butter
Olives
Avocadoes

We will count as carbohydrates and only as carbohydrates:

Fruits
Vegetables
Bread
Rice
Potatoes
Pasta
Sugar
Honey
Jam and jelly
Cakes, pies, cookies, candies, chocolate
Ice cream

Water, tea and coffee contain no calories and need not be counted. Alcohol does contain calories, and should be kept to a minimum if you want to get the most good out of your diet.

Once every item has been put into its correct category, we can proceed to the basic rule of the diet: at every meal, you are to take one portion of fat, two portions of protein, and either three or four portions of carbohydrate, depending on your taste.

There are three sub-rules:

1) Since a properly balanced diet should contain fat of both animal and vegetable origin, you will split up your

single portion of fat into two half portions, one animal (butter, cream), the other vegetable (margarine, oils, nuts, avocadoes, olives).

2) the two portions of protein should be divided in either of these two ways: one portion of meat, fish or eggs, and one of milk or milk products (cheese, yogurt, etc.); or, two portions of milk or milk products. You can give up meat anytime you feel like it, but your body needs milk regularly.

3) Your carbohydrate portions should be divided into one portion of raw vegetables or fruits; one portion of cooked vegetables or fruits; one portion of a starchy product—potatoes, bread, rice, cereal or pasta; and (optionally) one portion of a sweet product or dessert.

This sums up the whole diet. If you follow it, you are almost sure to be eating more or less correctly. Perhaps not at every meal, but if you vary menus in a normal way you will find that they average out and are giving you everything you need, in pretty much the proper proportions.

Simply repeat to yourself at the start of every meal.

½ animal fat
½ vegetable fat
1 meat protein
1 milk protein
1 raw fruit or vegetable
1 cooked fruit or vegetable
1 starch
1 sweet

Make up your mind that these, and these only, are what you are going to eat in the course of the meal. Check them off mentally, or on a piece of paper, as you eat each course. When you reach the limit, stop.

It should not be hard to stop, for there is a great deal of nourishment in a meal composed like this, and if you are

42

eating average-sized portions, there is no reason for your appetite not to be satisfied.

What, you may well have been itching to ask, do I mean by an average portion?

I am going to leave that entirely up to you.

The 1-2-4 diet can be put in a handy chart form, as follows:

Each square represents a portion to be taken daily.

Fats	Proteins	Carbohydrates
½ animal—butter or cream ½ vegetable—margarine, nuts, oils, mayonnaise, olives, avocadoes	1 meat, fish or eggs *or* 1 milk or milk product	1 raw fruit or vegetable
	1 milk or milk product	1 cooked fruit or vegetable
		1 starch—bread, cereal, potatoes, rice, pasta
		1 sweet—sugar, honey, chocolate, candy, desserts

Every time you are served food at a meal, put a check mark in the box at the lower righthand corner of each square. Make sure that you check each box at every meal, and make sure that you check it only once. Or if you check it twice, you must go on and check all the others.

Nothing is more annoying in most diets than being told that you must take exactly so many grams or ounces of such-and-such foods. You can, of course, carry a little scale around with you and put all your food on it before you eat it. But this is cumbersome and you may find it socially unacceptable. In addition, the figures given in diet books are based on averages, and we are none of us precisely average, so adjustments have to be made in the figures and that eats up more time and energy.

The purpose of this book is not to put you in a nutritional straitjacket, but to get you thinking in terms of proportions at all your meals.

So don't start out by worrying over the precise size of the hamburger you are going to have for lunch. You may be used to a three-ounce one, or a six-ounce one, you may for that matter be used to a 10-ounce sirloin steak. If it fits you, it counts as one meat-protein portion, and you can put down a little P on your pad to remind you that that part of your meal is past.

This is not a license to gorge yourself. I have to count on your being rational. A portion is not what you would like to have in a burst of euphoria, it is what you regard as a normal portion, sufficient for the normal appetite. If you eat a loaf of bread at every meal with a quarter of a pound of butter on it, if you insist on half an apple pie with three scoops of ice-cream for dessert you know very well—despite any attempts to talk yourself into believing the contrary—that there is something abnormal about your tastes; you are committing a nutritional crime and can only expect a nutritional disaster to follow. I don't mean that you cannot have a gargantuan feast from time to time. But if you really need that much food at every meal, something is very wrong with you, which needs more treatment than you can get out of this or any other book. You should see a doctor.

But within ordinary, reasonable limits, anything you regard as an ordinary, reasonable serving can be taken as a portion for purposes of the 1-2-4 diet.

Within those limits, the important thing is not the size of any individual portion. The important thing is to make sure that you get a portion of everything. In the old Mother Goose rhyme, Jack Sprat could eat no fat and his wife

44

could eat no lean. For the purpose of the rhyme, every-thing came out all right because they licked the platter clean. But you do not live in a Mother Goose world, and you must think of yourself and not of the platter. The Jack Sprat syndrome is exactly what you want to avoid at all costs. Both you and your spouse need both fat and lean. Your portions may be twice as big as those of your spouse, or vice versa. That is perfectly all right, as long as you both take the same number of portions, in the rhythm of 1-2-4 (or 1-2-3 as you prefer).

So much for the principles. Now let us try to put them into practice. First, let us take one of your present meals. Suppose you are used to a breakfast like this:

Orange juice
Cereal with
Cream and
Sugar
Bacon
Eggs
Toast (or pancakes) with
Butter and
Jam (or syrup)
Coffee with
Cream and
Sugar

This is a colossal breakfast by the standards of my coun-try, but the standards of my country are very defective on this point, and I am not opposed to your having a copious breakfast—far from it. What I do object to is the wildly unbalanced nature of this meal.

Let us check off each item:

The orange gives us one of our carbohydrates
    (the one for raw fruit or vegetable) (C)
The cereal gives us our starch carbohydrate (C)

45

The cream is an animal fat (F)
The sugar is our sweet carbohydrate (C)
The eggs are an animal protein (P)
So is the bacon (P)
The toast or pancakes are starch (C)
The butter is animal fat (F)
The jam is a sweet (C)
So is the sugar in the coffee (C)
The cream in the coffee is another fat (F)

If we total these up we get three F's, two P's, six C's. That is to say, three times as much fat and 50% more carbohydrate than is good for you. In addition, the distribution within each category is askew. You have two starch carbohydrates and three sweets, but not a single cooked vegetable or fruit. You have two meat proteins and no milk protein. You have three animal fats and not a single vegetable one.

Such a meal is made to order for putting on unwanted pounds, and it deprives you of some food elements your body needs.

Let us see how we can improve it by applying the 1-2-4 principle.

In the first place, let us cut down the excessive fat content. Replace the cream on the cereal by milk. This kills two birds with one stone, for we have suppressed an F and added the milk P which was missing.

Then we can suppress the cream in the coffee (it is a bad mixture anyway).

That leaves a single F, which is the butter, and if instead of the usual serving we make it half butter and half margarine, we have satisfactorily filled our fat quota.

The milk on the cereal has given us a milk P. We don't want two animal P's, so we suppress either the bacon or the eggs. (Or, if you prefer, we can cut the serving in half: instead of two eggs and four strips of bacon, make it one egg and two strips.)

Now for the carbohydrates. We have one raw C with the orange juice, and that is fine. We need a cooked C, and so we should add something like stewed prunes or apple-sauce. We have two starches, and we have to get rid of one of them.

If we keep the cereal, and get rid of the toast, we may be in a little trouble, because what then are you going to do with your butter-margarine portion? You could put it in oatmeal, but I don't see it going very well with something like cornflakes. If worse comes to worst, you can just drop your fat ration out of breakfast entirely and increase it a bit at both lunch and dinner. I would try to do as little of such shifting as possible, for all your meals should be of approximately equal size, to spread your energy supply evenly through the day. But the rule is not meant to be ty-rannical, and you can make minor adjustments like this anytime you want.

If you choose toast, there is no problem. You have half your serving with butter and half with margarine or pea-nut butter.

As far as the sweet carbohydrate is concerned, you have the choice between sugar on your cereal (or jam or honey on your toast) and sugar in your coffee.

If you have chosen toast instead of cereal, you are short one P, for the milk. You can take a glass of milk instead, or a piece of cheese if your tastes run that way.

This menu is open to infinite variation, and you can ex-ercise your ingenuity on it. You might try blueberry pan-cakes with butter and margarine and maple syrup, for in-stance, giving you three C's (starch and cooked fruit and sweet) and one F. Round it out with half a grapefruit (raw C), ham or eggs or half a slice of ham and one egg (meat), and a glass of milk (milk P), and you have a fine 1-2-4 meal which conforms to my principles and should satisfy your appetite.

Let us now move on from breakfast to the midday meal. We started our breakfasts with an example that was positively swollen with unwanted fats and carbohydrates. Let us now go to the other extreme.

Too many people in the rush of modern business life take too little time for lunch and cut down the meal drastically both to save time and in the hope of cutting down their weight. You will lose more time in fatigue caused by insufficient nourishment, and as for weight control, that can be an illusion. It is a common sight to see a secretary rush out of her office, down to a lunch counter and order something like this:

> A fresh fruit salad (C) with
> Cottage cheese (P)
> Iced tea (–)

Even if she puts a dab of mayonnaise on it, which we may mark ½ F, our totals are only ½ F, one P, one C, which is a pitiful excuse for a meal. It is short in every single requirement, and it is not well designed for reducing either, for fruits are chock-full of carbohydrates, hence of calories.

There is no need to turn this into a heavy meal in order to balance it. It is perfectly possible to have a light lunch which won't make you feel groggy in the afternoon, and yet give you the kind of variety you need.

Try, for instance:

> A tuna fish salad (the tuna is animal protein and the green vegetables chopped with it provide our raw carbohydrate) (PC)
>
> Toast (starch) (C)
>
> Butter (half what you would usually take)—animal fat (½ F)
>
> The same amount of margarine—vegetable fat (½ F)

A side order of vegetables or a cooked fruit (C)

A glass of milk or a serving of cottage cheese (P)

A dessert or a couple of lumps of sugar in your tea (if you take the dessert, use a sugar substitute in your beverage) (C)

This gives us a total of one F, two P's, four C's. Even if you cut it down by suppressing the dessert or sugar (counting 1-2-3 instead of 1-2-4) you will still have a meal substantial enough to see you through the afternoon, and it will spare you those violent urges for chocolate bars or cherry pies that can come over you at about 4:00 P.M.

Here is another way you could make up a light lunch: try two small sandwiches, one with cream cheese and olives, the other with egg salad. We now have:

Bread (starch) (C)

Egg (animal protein) (P)

Olives (probably not very many
so we can call this half a fat ration) (½ F)

Cream cheese (milk protein) (P)

Lettuce, pickles, or whatever other vegetables
are mixed with the egg (C)

Applesauce (cooked fruit) (C)

With a little bit of cream (½ F)

The totals here are one F, two P's, and three C's. Sugar in your tea or coffee will turn this 1-2-3 meal into a 1-2-4. If there was mayonnaise in your egg salad, you would have to count another ½ F and thus go over your ration. You would then suppress your vegetable fat in the evening.

49

Take another bad example: it is common to see some-one order a single, or a double-decker, hamburger sand-wich and a cup of coffee and let it go at that.

If it is a double-decker, we have a count of two P's which is a mistake to begin with, since both protein por-tions are meat and one of them should be milk.

The bread of the sandwich gives us one C. Even if there is some lettuce and tomato thrown in, this gives us only one extra C, for a total of two P's and two C's.

With such a meal you are eating more protein than your body can efficiently handle, and not enough of the other essentials. It would be much healthier to order a meal like this:

An order of chopped steak	(P)
Spinach or string beans	(C)
Mashed potatoes	(C)
With a little butter	(½ F)
Some lettuce	(C)
With a little oil	(½ F)
And vinegar (which we needn't count, any more than we need count a bit of mustard or other con-diment you might want to put on your meat)	
A piece of apple pie	(C)
With a piece of cheese	(P)
Black coffee (which also does not count)	

Here we have one F, two P's, and four C's. This is more varied and interesting than the simple hamburger, and is a far better support for you during the hours to come.

Of course you don't always have to have a light lunch. You may be invited out to a fancy restaurant and have a wide variety of tempting dishes to choose from. You could start with:

Artichoke hearts (cooked) (C)

With a little olive oil (vegetable fat) (½ F)

And vinegar (which we don't count)

and go on to:

any meat or fish that strikes your fancy (P)

With the chef's favorite sauce (½ F)
(made with butter and so an animal fat). If you are serious about dieting, you will be better off without the sauce, because cooked fat is harder to digest than raw. If you can do it without hurting the chef's feelings, I suggest you take your meat or fish grilled, and your animal fat ration in the form of butter on your bread or potatoes)

Bread (or potatoes, or rice, or spaghetti) (C)

A piece of fine cheese (P)

Some fresh fruit (C)

Sugar in your coffee if your wish (C)

This provides one F, two P's, and three or four C's. And you have a wholesome and satisfying meal.
Try this menu for your evening meal:

Vegetable soup (C)

An omelet (cooked in a Teflon pan with no grease)
(P)

A salad (C)

With a little dressing (½ F)

Bread or toast	(C)
With a little butter	(½ F)
Cheese or milk	(P)
Cookies or cake or sugar in your tea or coffee	(C)

This results in one F, two P's and four C's.

I think this is enough to give you the general idea. You can go on indefinitely switching foods around, so long as you keep to the 1-2-4 proportion.

Try to visualize your day's food as a whole, so that you won't overdo any one item. If you have potatoes at lunch, for example, don't have them again at night; make sure you get green vegetables. And vice versa.

The important thing is to keep to the proportions. Every one of those F's, P's and C's is essential for the proper functioning of your body. Counting up to four at every meal is not too high a price to pay for making sure you get them.

Remember you are allowed only one portion in each category. You can't have both cereal and toast for breakfast (unless you are willing to cut each serving in half) because they are both starchy C's. You can't have both potatoes and rice at dinner, for the same reason. You shouldn't have lobster and steak at the same meal, both animal proteins—you will pay a fortune for the lobster, and all those extra proteins will pass through your system without doing you a bit of good. You can have apple pie, or you can have ice cream, but you can't have apple pie à la mode.

Suppose you are really hungry, though, and you have an uncontrollable urge for apple pie à la mode. Or you want two orders of anything else on the menu. Do you have to get up from the table bent over with hunger?

No, I will allow you to double up. Triple up, for that matter. There are occasions in life when you deserve a really big, soul-satisfying meal.

But I will quickly add a condition. If you want to double up on one dish, you must double up on all. Apple pie à la mode? All right, but in that case you will also take two orders of meat, two of milk, two of raw fruit or vegetable, two of cooked fruit or vegetable, two of fat. You double up across the board or not at all.

I won't blame you for being skeptical when you hear this. Most people are. If I ate all that at every meal, doctor, I'd grow as big as a house, they say.

Well, of course. If you eat a mountain of food at every meal, you will get pretty mountainous yourself in fairly short order. But if you are a normal human being, the chances are overwhelming that you won't do any such thing.

I treat obese men, women and children in my clinic every day. They are still, fortunately, only a small minority of the population, though bad eating habits increase their numbers shockingly year by year. And only a small minority (less than 15%) of these patients are the kind of people who eat everything, who cannot stop shovelling all kinds of food into their stomachs. Such people have a very serious illness, and the treatment is long, complex and uncertain. They have to be given pills to depress their appetites, and these pills can have a bad effect on their nerves. Then they literally have to be taught to eat all over again, and this is a very difficult task.

I assume that you are not in this small class of unfortunates. (If you are, look for professional advice at once.) As long as you are not, I am sure that doubling up on your portions once in a while will not do you any harm.

The reason is that the average person does not get fat by eating too much of everything he sees. He gets fat by eating too much of one or two categories of food. He gorges on candy, or on bread and butter, or on beer, and he neglects other foods in the process. There is nothing intrinsically wrong with candy, with bread and butter, even with beer in moderation (though it can produce gas in your stomach). But they are easy to overindulge in, because they do not satisfy your appetite the way protein-rich food does. If you forget about the principle of proportions and keep on stuffing in foods like these, you will inevitably get fat. But if you keep to the proportions, if you keep your diet in balance, you won't feel the need to stuff them in.

Your body may well be willing to accept a double order of potatoes. But it is unlikely to put up with a whole double meal as a steady diet. So you may take your double meal on rare occasions and need not feel guilty about it. The principle of balanced proportions will see you through in the long run.

Do not feel guilty, either, if any given one of your 1-2-4 meals seems particularly high—or skimpy—in caloric count. There is no need to count calories at all while you are following it—though of course if you are so inclined you can do so, using the table you will find in a later chapter—so long as you keep varying your menus from day to day. It is highly desirable to vary them, because if you get bored with eating the same damned thing day in and day out you will be tempted to cut down on some of your portions and you may lose something vital in the process. As long as you do change around from day to day, it is likely that things will even out in the end, and that over a week or a month you will be getting approximately the right number of calories, distributed in approximately the right proportions.

If so, your weight will cease to be a problem; it will take care of itself.

III
Some ABC's of Nutrition

The 1-2-4 diet is simple and fun to follow, and easy to apply in most situations in your daily life. It can by itself improve your eating habits and thus improve your health.

You may, however, want more. You may be interested in preparing for some activity which is going to call on all your resources and for which you want to be prepared in the best possible way. This activity need not be an athletic competition, it can be any crucial moment in your life. I will refer to it as the Event.

To get ready for the Event, you will want a more detailed and more carefully planned ration than the useful but imprecise one you can construct by using the 1-2-4 principle. I have worked out such a ration through long studies in cooperation with some 400 picked athletes. This was the regular diet which enabled them to perform best and most consistently.

It will naturally take a little more time and effort to follow this regimen than the 1-2-4. But it is not difficult. Its central principle is simple indeed:

The food you eat in the course of any day, no matter what quantity is required for your particular body, should be divided into:

15% proteins
30% fats
55% carbohydrates

The closer you can stick to these proportions, the better you will look, feel and act. This is the ideal combination to get the most out of the energy potential of your body.

I will show you in detail how to translate these ideal proportions into meals which are appetizing as well as nutritious and which will allow you to eat at least a bit of almost all the foods you like.

But first, I think you will be more motivated to follow the diet if you understand the reasons for it. I will try to show you why these 15-30-55 proportions are so important, and to do that I will give you a brief review of some of the basic principles, the ABC's of human nutrition, not to burden you with information but to help you see why I give you the advice I do. This advice is not a tablet of law brought down from Mount Sinai, but plain common sense based on recognized facts about the human body, and if you are acquainted with them it will make it easier for you to follow this or any other diet.

The first thing to know about your digestive system is that it is marvelously constructed, marvelously complex.

Consider a very simple daily event: you eat a piece of bread.

As far as you consciously are concerned, all you do is put it in your mouth, give it a few perfunctory bites, swallow it, feel it go down with a more or less pleasant sensation, and that is the end of the matter. You are only aware of the subsequent process if something goes wrong and your innards call attention to themselves by growling or sputtering or doubling you up with pain.

But this subsequent process which takes place almost totally outside of your awareness is a wondrous piece of work. Here is a simplified account of what happens:

The basic component of bread, outside of a great deal of water and a little protein, is starch. Starch is a complex sugar molecule which cannot be directly absorbed by the body but has to be broken down into the simpler form of maltose. Some of this is done in your mouth by your saliva which turns the starch of your bread successively into:

Soluble starch
Erythodextrin
α-acrodextrin
β-acrodextrin

and finally maltose.

Not all of it, however; depending on how hard and how fast you chew, a certain percentage of the bread is not dissolved by your saliva but goes down to your stomach as pure starch. There the stomach enzymes will work on it, and if your digestive system is working properly, all the starch in your bread will eventually arrive in your small intestine in the form of pure maltose. (If it is not working right, some will pass into the colon, which is not specialized for breaking it down into maltose, and the results will be dyspepsia and flatulence.)

In the small intestine, maltose has to be broken down further so that it can pass through the intestinal wall into capillaries of the bloodstream. This is done by enzymes which transform the maltose into glucose. Ferried by the bloodstream to the liver it is again transformed into glycogen, a form in which it can be conserved and held in readiness for future use (just the way we put food in the freezer). It is stocked both in the liver and (ferried again through the blood) in the muscles, and when the body needs to expend energy it calls on these reserves. The amount of glycogen you can stock at any one time is strictly limited—no more than 500 grams or so. If there is more glucose in your digestive tract than you can stock as glycogen, the rest will be stocked in a different way—as fat—and this is the most common cause for putting on weight.

Through the action of agents created in the liver, enzymes called phosphorylase α and β, glycogen passes successively through the following phases:

Phosphoric-1-glucose ester
Phosphoric-6-glucose ester
Fructo-pyranose-6-phosphoric ester
Fructo-pyranose-di-phosphoric ester

At this point, mixed with TDA (triphosphoric adenosyne acid) which is derived from other foods you have eaten, like meat, it becomes DPA (diphosphoric adenosyne acid), then phosphoro-3-glycinic acid, and then pyruvic acid.

At this point it is ready to enter into the combustion process which takes place as you contract your muscles. This process is known as the Krebs isocitric cycle. In each stage of this cycle the remnants of what was your piece of bread loses molecules containing carbon, oxygen or hydrogen and becomes successively

Isoconitric acid
Isocitric acid
Oxalysuccinic acid
A-cetoglutanic acid
Succinic acid
Fumaric acid
Malic acid
Oxaloacetic acid,

after which it becomes pyruvic acid again, and the whole Krebs cycle is repeated till every last drop of the original glycogen is used up and transformed into energy. If you want to keep on using your muscles then you will have to get some more fuel to them in a hurry. Otherwise they will lose their elasticity, and you will begin to suffer from paleness, sweat, weakness and hunger.

This is the only example of technical detail I will burden you with. You need not remember all those chemical names, but I do want to give you an idea of the extraordinary complexity of the energy-consuming engine that is your body. It is an engine which has been finely tuned for you by Nature, and that is why I insist that our clumsy human theories should tamper with it as little as possible.

Your body knows pretty well what it wants in food, and when, and tries to let you know by the mechanisms of hunger and appetite.

Hunger is a purely physical phenomenon. When your engine is running short of the fuel it needs to keep going, a signal is sent out by your hypothalamus. It is like the red light that goes on in the dashboard of some cars to let you know you are running out of gas.

But after all, you are not an automobile engine, and eating is a far more complicated business than driving up to a gas pump at periodic intervals.

Eating is a social, an emotional and a symbolic act as well as a physical one. It is based on a physical need, but the particular forms it takes, the content of your meals, the times and places you choose to eat them, are all—like your table manners—largely a matter of conditioning. Most of the conditioning is done in childhood and by the time we are grown up it is so much a part of ourselves that we regard it as a law of Nature and feel incomprehension if not hostility when we meet people with habits very different from our own.

There is, when you come down to it, no law of Nature

59

which says that we have to have three and only three meals a day. But most of us have been brought up that way, and intend to live and die that way, and if someone like Dr. R. C. Hutchinson comes along with what he calls statistical proof that we would work more efficiently if we took six meals a day, we don't pay him the slightest attention.

Even when there is a genuine interest in exotic ways, the pull of upbringing is likely to prove stronger in the long run. Again and again I have seen athletes come to the Olympic village full of curiosity about the diet of their rivals from strange and distant lands. Often they shop around, experiment a little; sometimes they become fascinated by exotic dishes. I have seen Western athletes develop a passion for the spicy rice dishes of the Far East, French athletes discover the delights of the copious Anglo-Saxon breakfast with its ham and eggs. But after a few days, these passions die, the Occidentals go back to their meat and potatoes, the French go back (over my bitter protests) to a cup of coffee and a croissant for breakfast.

We tell ourselves that we choose our meals because we like the taste of certain foods and dislike that of others. And, of course, this is a serious consideration, which should always be kept in mind in planning your diet; everybody comes naturally by certain likes and dislikes. But not so much as you may think. A goodly number of those likes and dislikes are not triggered by anything in your physical makeup, they are purely cultural phenomena. If you were told that the delicious meat patty you just ate was made of earthworms, adders' tongues and minced cockroaches, you would probably get sick, just like a pious Jew or Moslem who was told he had eaten pork, or a Hindu who was told he had eaten cow. Yet, from the strictly physical point of view, all these foods are equally full of proteins and equally nutritious.

I can vividly recall, in the dining hall at the winter Olympics in Grenoble in 1968, being intrigued by the elaborate ceremonial with which a huge covered bowl was brought in to the Korean skaters at a table nearby. They were in a state of ecstasy when the bowl was uncovered, and my friends and I couldn't resist walking over to see what was the cause of all this rapture. One whiff was enough to make a strong—or at least a strong Western European—man fall over. It was a dish of fermented green cabbage leaves, and would have put any of our men out of competition at once. But it seemed to do the Koreans no harm; they won a championship.

Some food is eaten for purely symbolic reasons. I know many men who believe that the blood dripping from a nice rare steak is specially rich in all sorts of values that will strengthen their muscles and increase their virility; they are sometimes impolitely skeptical when a doctor like myself assures them that the nutritional value of their steak is no greater and no less than that of an equivalent amount of mackerel.

(Actually, the red juice that comes out of rare meat is little more than colored water. I have known many poor children who were fed gallons of this stuff in the vain hope that it would fill their bodies with good red blood.)

Let us disregard all these subjective elements for the time being and stick to the bare physical necessities; what your body needs to stay alive and keep working efficiently.

First, to stay alive. If you never moved a muscle all day long, if you were in a state of hibernation, you would still need to maintain a minimum level of largely unconscious activity which guarantees that you are alive and not dead: your heart must beat, your lungs must breathe, blood must circulate through your arteries and veins, your glands must maintain certain secretions. You need some caloric intake for all that. And you need some more to replace the wear and tear on your organism, the waste products which pass out in sweat, breath, urine or feces every day.

All these basic requirements come in the average healthy adult to about 1,500 calories a day (up to 10% more or less if you are bigger or smaller than the average—5'9" and 154 pounds for men, 5'4" and 128 pounds for women).

Perhaps this is the time to say exactly what is meant by calorie, a word often taken in vain. A calorie is a unit of energy; it indicates the amount necessary to raise the temperature of one kilogram of water from 16 to 17 degrees Centigrade under normal atmospheric conditions. It is not an ideal measure of bodily energy, for though calories *do* count, they do not all count alike, and merely toting up the calories you eat in the course of a day can be misleading and even dangerous as well as time consuming. As I continually tell my patients, you don't eat calories, you eat steak and green peas and apple pie, and I urge them to think in portions of these.

Nevertheless, calories are the most common and familiar unit we have, and I will go on referring to them in this book. It is just as well to have a general idea of the caloric value of the foods you eat—not so much the total number of calories as the number brought in the form of proteins, fats and carbohydrates respectively—so long as you don't get obsessed with the subject. Count if you wish, but as I have shown in the last chapter and will show again in the next, it is perfectly possible to eat in a sensible, well-balanced, weight-controlling way without ever counting a single calorie.

Let us assume then that you need around 1,500 calories just to keep you alive (your basal metabolism). Over and above this, you need another, indeterminate amount to provide the energy for whatever activities you perform, whatever muscles you move, during the course of the day.

Figuring out exactly what this amounts to is not as easy as most diet books would have you believe. It is easy to draw up charts of averages and tell you, this is exactly how many calories you need in the course of a day, but the averages may have nothing to do with your own particular case. It is relatively easy to study individuals performing particular physical actions and determine how much energy they burn up in the process. It has been shown, for example, that a tailor burns up on the average 44 calories an hour above his basal metabolism, a shoemaker 90, a woodchopper 388, a weight-lifter 450, a long-distance runner 750, a downhill skier 960, and so on. It has even been determined that the calorie output per square meter of body surface is 1.4 for a saxophonist, 1.5 for a bagpipe player, and 2 for a pianist.

These figures are fascinating, but what do they have to do with your own particular needs?

Nutrition is not a matter of simple arithmetic, though many nutritionists like to think so. I have heard it seriously argued that since 100 grams of glucose releases just the amount of energy that is spent in swimming for one hour, the best way to prepare for an hour's swim is to swallow 100 grams of sugar. By the same logic the best way to prepare for a 10-hour swim would be to swallow a kilogram of sugar, which even a nutritionist would find unpleasant, if not impossible.

Similarly, there is no simple one-to-one relation between the number of calories you eat and the number of pounds you weigh. I have had under my care in the hospital a man who kept his weight at more than 300 pounds though he ate no more than 2,000 calories a day, and I have known an 18-year-old swimmer who took in the colossal total of 12,000 calories a day without getting fat.

These of course are extreme cases. But everyone's case is special. In the long run, if you want to know your caloric output, you will have to figure it out for yourself. You can do this roughly in a period when you are following a fairly uniform diet and your weight seems to be keeping steady. You can add up, with the help of the figures you will find in Chapter V, the total number of calories in the food you eat in the course of any particular day. Subtract the 1,500 (plus or minus up to 10% depending on your size) calories for your basal metabolism. (To be technically correct, you should also subtract a few other calories for such things as the energy you spend keeping your body temperature constant, but under most conditions this is negligible—modern man uses clothes, central heating and air conditioning instead of his own autoregulatory processes for this purpose.)

Once you have made the subtraction, you have a figure which gives a reasonably accurate count of what you expend in the way of energy in your daily activities.

The variation from individual to individual can be enormous. For an athlete in training, the hourly caloric expenditure can vary between 100 and 300, at the moment of competition it can go up to 500 and beyond.

The precise figure obviously depends on many factors, including body build, nervous tension, skill (an awkward player expends more energy in waste motion and therefore needs more calories than a well-coordinated one).

Let us assume, for purposes of this discussion, that you are an average healthy man or woman engaging in some form of strenuous physical activity every day, and that you will need 3,200 calories per day (for men) or 2,700 (for women) to keep in proper shape for these activities.

Now to see how to distribute these calories through your daily meals.

Let me repeat the principle: your intake of calories every day should consist of:

15% protein
30% fat
55% carbohydrate

I will take up each category in turn.

PROTEINS

The word protein comes from the Greek *protos* meaning first, and it is easy to see why the early scientists who first identified and named these compounds chose to emphasize their primacy. They are the indispensable food. We could hobble along without carbohydrates or without fats, but without proteins we would quickly die.

Proteins are the basic building blocks of any living organism, and are essential to all the principal body functions: nutrition, growth, reproduction. The protein molecule is the substratum of every living cell, and has its role to play in almost everything your body does, from the formation of contractile tissue in the muscles to the building of hormones, enzymes, antibodies.

The proteins in the food we eat are broken down in our digestive tract into amino-acids. These can, exceptionally, when the body is short of sugar, be changed into sugar and burned for energy, by the process known as neoglycogenesis. But this can be done only to a limited extent. Your body needs the proteins you eat to maintain its own structure, and under the best of circumstances can spare only enough to provide about one-eighth of your daily energy requirements. It cannot spare any more because the lack of protein in your cells would be worse than the fatigue, or even collapse, resulting from lack of fuel for energy.

The main, the vital function of proteins is plastic-building and repairing the cells of the body.

For the purpose of building and repairing human body cells, proteins of animal origin (meat, fish, milk, eggs) are superior to those of vegetable origin (those derived from bread, rice, potatoes, beans, etc.), and consequently they should make up the majority of your 15% daily ration.

I realize that this statement will arouse the ire of many who believe that eating meat is sinful as well as harmful.

If their prejudice extends only to meat, or to meat and

65

fish, I have no serious quarrel with them. I won't even quarrel with the tender-hearted who consider that eating an egg is the equivalent of murdering a little chicken, but they must at least drink milk even if it has been brutally squeezed from an animal body. All these foods—meat, fish, eggs, milk—are equally valuable as sources of protein. They are in fact pretty much interchangeable at your meals, except that while you can always replace meat by milk, you must never totally suppress milk from your diet because it contains calcium in considerable quantities and meat does not.

When it comes to radical vegetarians who reject everything from the animal kingdom, including milk and cheese, I am firmly convinced they are asking for trouble. The reason is simple: animal proteins are a richer and more reliable source of the eight or so amino acids which are considered essential because the human body cannot fabricate them itself but must get them in the form of food. They come ready-made, so to speak, in animal protein, available every time you eat meat, fish, eggs, or milk. To duplicate the same amino acids from food derived from vegetables, you need a complicated and scientifically balanced dose of soybeans, wheat, corn and other products, which is not always easy to manufacture or procure. If you do not get the right dose of the essential amino acids, you are laying yourself open to premature aging and lowered resistance to infection, because your body simply does not replace itself adequately as it wears out.

I am aware of the experiments made by reputable men of science which are supposed to prove that a meatless diet is beneficial for physical effort. Irving Fisher, for example, once asked a small group of vegetarians to hold their right arms out straight. They could hold them for impressive periods of time, one going to 200 minutes. He tested a group of carnivorous subjects too, and they were pitiful in comparison: they let their arms fall after a lapse of, on the average, only 22 minutes.

One of his vegetarians could do as many as 927 knee-bends, while his best meat-eater could do only 383.

These results, and similar tests conducted by Iotyko and Kipiano, look impressive enough. But they leave out of account one very important consideration: just what was the nutritional state of the subjects before the tests began? Were Fisher's carnivores typical of other carnivores? Were they *well-fed* carnivores?

I decided to duplicate Fisher's experiments in my own laboratory. I found my own groups of vegetarians and of heavy meat-eaters, and had them perform the same motions as in Fisher's experiments. The differences were far less dramatic than his (in the knee-bend, for example, the vegetarians did between 198 and 322, the carnivores between 177 and 219. Still, there was a difference and one that seemed clearly unfavorable to the meat-eaters.

But I pushed the experiment a little further. I asked all my subjects to change their diets temporarily and follow my 15-30-55 proportions, with the 15% of protein coming for the most part from meat sources. It was not easy to persuade the vegetarians to eat any meat at all, even in the pursuit of scientific truth, and almost as difficult to persuade the others to give up some of their juicy red steaks. But they finally agreed, and after three months of carefully supervising their menus, I tested them again. This time everybody's performance was improved. The first (ex-vegetarian) group now did between 209 and 374 knee-bends, the other group between 216 and 282. The moral would seem to be that while a vegetarian diet may help you to perform physical feats more than one that is too rich in meat, both are inferior to a well-balanced over-all diet.

Now let us see what is the best way of getting 15% of your daily calories in high quality proteins. Assuming a daily intake of 3,200 calories for a man (2,700 for a woman), that would make 480 (405).

(Remember throughout this and all other discussions of

daily totals that your own individual needs may be greater or less, so that all figures would have to be adjusted accordingly. My figures of 3,200 and 2,700 for daily caloric
intake are on the high side; they assume a fair amount of
vigorous physical activity every day. If you are not getting that, then my figures will have to be scaled down by
10 or 20% or even more. You alone can determine what
your daily total of food should be. I can only tell you how
to divide it up.)

We have then a daily total of 480 (405) calories to come
from proteins every day. Since we want a majority of
these to come from animal proteins, I recommend eating
250 grams (9 ounces) of meat every day, divided as you
wish between red meat and poultry, and replaced two or
three times a week by fish (for the sake of variety) and at
one meal a week by liver (for the sake of the vitamins A
and B complex); 350 grams (12 ounces) of milk every day;
50 grams (2 ounces) of cheese every day; 4 or 5 eggs a
week. As you can figure out from the tables that will be
given in Chapter V, this will produce something like 350
calories. The rest of the 480 will come from bread and
other foods which you will be eating primarily for their
contribution in carbohydrates, and which we will discuss
later.

The 15% figure represents an ideal balance between
too much and too little protein.

If you eat significantly less than 15% your body will
run down as it fails to replace worn-out cell matter. You
will lose in both physical and mental efficiency and lay
yourself open to trouble in your liver, kidneys and endocrine glands. If you stopped eating protein altogether,
your body would start devouring the protein in its own
cells and before it got halfway through you would
die.

Eating too much protein has less dramatic consequences. You cannot possibly die of too much protein;
however, you can suffer serious inconveniences which

can interfere with physical activity. You may pile up urea, uric acid and ammonia in your blood, which can tire you out, weaken your tendons, and cause headaches and high blood pressure. If your protein intake goes above 20% of the total, your body will be faced with a surplus which it cannot use for maintaining or repairing tissues. It will have to burn up this surplus, creating unnecessary heat, sometimes even causing a fever, or harming you with left-over toxins.

In general therefore, you should be careful to keep your protein ration from going much higher than 15%. (Another consideration is that protein-rich foods generally cost a good deal more than others.)

There are exceptional cases, however, when you not only can but should increase your protein intake. At certain periods, notably adolescence and pregnancy, the body is building new tissue so rapidly that it needs more protein. For the pregnant woman, this new tissue is her baby, for the adolescent it is the expansion of limbs and organs all over. The athlete in training is in a certain sense in the same situation: building muscles means creating new tissue.

If, then, you are in training, and for the limited time when you are actually building up muscles, you may increase your protein intake (preferably animal) by 50 or even 100%.

Be very careful if you do so, however, and do not suddenly start piling extra proteins into your system. There will be a strain on your liver and kidneys handling the extra amino acids, and if you overdo it you will create toxins in your blood which will cause fatigue and counteract all the benefit you expect to get from the new muscle tissue. Be sure to drink plenty of water to keep clearing the toxins out. A good rule of thumb is to drink an extra glass of water for every 50 grams of meat you add to your daily diet. And be sure to stop the extra protein after two or three weeks.

Now let us turn to the second main component of our food.

FAT

Like protein, fat comes from both animal and vegetable sources. But unlike what we observed about protein, the vegetable fats are better for you than the animal, and should be favored in your daily diet.

Prime sources of animal fat are butter, cream, lard; and there are varying amounts of fat in all meat, fish, whole milk and eggs.

Vegetable fat comes primarily from oils squeezed out of plants like olive, peanut, corn, safflower; and oily fruits and nuts like olives, avocadoes, almonds, peanuts, walnuts, etc.

Both categories have a place in your diet. The reason you should emphasize vegetable fats is that they can supply you, as animal fats cannot, with certain essential fatty acids which your body needs and cannot synthesize from other foods. If you run short of these acids, you may develop eye and skin trouble, and suffer from severe lack of energy.

I do not, however, go along with some overenthusiastic authorities who have recommended giving up animal fat entirely. For one thing, it would mean giving up all your present consumption of meat, fish, eggs, milk and cheese; and living on a diet of skimmed milk and fat-free cottage cheese is neither particularly appetizing nor particularly healthy. As far as butter is concerned, it is far too good a source of vitamin A to be dispensed with entirely.

Animal fats tend to be more saturated (i.e., contain more hydrogen atoms) than vegetable. The more saturated a fat is, the harder it is for the organism to use it; it takes more work to get it properly absorbed.

Animal fats also contain more cholesterol, and you

70

have heard often enough that cholesterol is a killer. It can be indeed a killer if you stock inordinate amounts in your blood: it can provoke the clogging up of your arteries by sticking to their walls. And arterial disease is one of the scourges of modern times. You had better make sure that your cholesterol count is not too high before you make any dietary plans whatever. If it does turn out to be too high, you will naturally have to follow your doctor's orders, and he will undoubtedly tell you to cut out animal fats as much as possible; but as long as your count is normal, there is no reason to give up this satisfying and nutritious source of energy.

Cholesterol is, after all, not in itself a poison; it is in fact an essential part of the hormones necessary for every physical effort. Athletes put a great strain on their hormones in the intensity of competition, and thus have a particular need not to run short of cholesterol. You have to strike a balance. Even if your cholesterol count is satisfactory at present, it is not a good idea to switch to an exclusive diet of eggs fried in butter. Your count may go up dramatically the next time you are tested.

There are many misconceptions about fat, the most dangerous of which is that fat is not very important, that we can do without it, it is only surplus weight we have to carry around with us. This is quite untrue. Fat has a most important role to play in fueling your body functions.

It has by far the highest energy potential among the three main components of your food. A gram of fat produces nine calories of energy when it is burned up in your body, while a gram of carbohydrate or protein produces only four.

And besides being a potent source of energy, it plays a vital role in many of your most vital functions. Almost 60%, for example, of the nourishment for the heart muscle whose steady beat keeps you alive comes from fatty acids.

In addition to the adipocytes, the specific fat cells

71

which are scattered all through your body, there is a quantity of fat in every single cell you have, in muscle, bone, brain, skin or wherever, and this is a quantity your body cannot do without; it needs them among other things to transport the fat-soluble vitamins A, D, E and K which are necessary to your survival.

This fat which is so necessary for our existence has to be supplied by the food we eat. If you don't eat enough fat to do the job directly, carbohydrates in your food will obligingly transform themselves into fat to give you what it needs. But this is a roundabout way of doing things, and if you misjudge the quantity of carbohydrates you need you are apt to get both dyspepsia and a rubber tire around your stomach. No one has cared to experiment on what the effect of a totally fat-free diet would be on humans. In rats, it stunts growth, develops skin lesions and problems of vision, and disturbs the functioning of the reproductive system.

The right proportion of fat in your daily caloric intake is 30%. This may strike you as a good deal, after you have been told in my 1-2-4 diet in the last chapter to take only one fat portion per meal, to two of protein and four of carbohydrate. The explanation is simple. A gram of fat produces nine calories, or more than twice as much as a gram of protein or carbohydrate, which produces only four, and therefore a little fat goes a long way.

Furthermore, a good deal of fat comes to you in disguise, so to speak, in foods where you do not ordinarily think of it as hiding—oysters for instance, 25% of whose calories come from fat; or eggs (16%). Even fruits and green vegetables have minute quantities of fat.

In fact, well over half of your 30% daily ration will come in other foods, and the amount of specifically fatty food you have to take is quite limited. This is just as well, because the more fat you try to get down at a time, the harder it is to digest.

Assuming a daily caloric intake of 3,200 calories, you will not need more than about 50 to 60 grams. Because the major part of this should be in vegetable fat, it can be divided as follows:

    2 tablespoons of butter
    2 tablespoons of vegetable oil
    1 tablespoon of margarine

Note that it takes more time to digest fats, especially cooked fats, than other foods. They may take up to eight hours to be completely assimilated. Therefore, it is best to keep consumption of fats down to a minimum before any violent physical effort. Fried foods should be avoided any time you are in training, and are absolutely not to be touched at any moment when the Event is approaching.

Some authorities claim that you need more fat when you are in a cold climate. Some mountain climbers and Arctic explorers have reported an almost uncontrollable urge for fat, others have not. The medical evidence is mixed. I personally am of the opinion that there is no need to eat more fat in very cold weather if you are wearing enough clothes to keep you warm. Only when your body has to come into direct contact with the elements without protective covering, as in swimming the English Channel or the St. Lawrence River, or in sports like canoeing and waterskiing where you may be in for unexpected spills in unpleasantly chilly water, would I recommend a slight increase in your fat ration. I will take up this problem later, when I speak of the special dietary requirements for different sports.

But in general I would say stick to the 30%; it is your ideal fat ration.

CARBOHYDRATE

The principal function of carbohydrates is to provide you with glucose, a sugar which your body can quickly and efficiently turn into muscular energy.

The primary role of carbohydrates in furnishing energy to the body has been recognized since the day in 1867 when two Swiss doctors named Fick and Wiscelenius climbed the Faulhorn. Up to that time it had been generally believed that our muscles were directly nourished by eating other animal muscles, like meat, i.e., protein. The two doctor-alpinists kept analyzing their urine as they climbed the mountain, and discovered that their bodies were not losing any amino acids. They deduced that proteins played no part in the energy-producing process. We know today that they were wrong because they didn't keep up their good work long enough. If they had tested their urine after they came down, they would have discovered a definite loss. But basically the doctors were right and they turned subsequent research in the right direction: it is not proteins but carbohydrates which form the primary source of muscular energy.

Like many a true word, this one is often pushed too far. A popular superstition has grown up, one that has done much harm over the years, which says that sugar equals energy; therefore, eating sugar will give you all the energy you need. I was appalled at the Tokyo Olympics of 1964 to see athletes from many continents in thrall to this superstition: they would scoop up handfuls of sugar lumps from the dining room tables and go off to munch them all day long. Perhaps the fact that sugar was free in the Olympic village got them excited. At all events, the results could be disastrous. Athletes put on weight before my eyes; they developed boils. My solution for the French team was to replace sugar lumps with powdered sugar in the bowls on the tables. They found it less tempting to fill their pockets with this somewhat messy product, and the alarming symptoms quickly disappeared.

A good 55% of your daily caloric intake should be in the form of carbohydrates. Almost all of this will go directly into energy.

Your liver and muscles can stock from 300 to 500 grams, representing 1,200 to 2,000 calories, or a little less than two-thirds of a day's normal needs. Any extra carbohydrates which do not go directly into energy or into this reserve stock are turned into fat and stored in your fatty tissue—a good reason for not letting your carbohydrate consumption get out of hand.

There are other reasons for not eating too many carbohydrates:

1) Starches are slower to digest than most other foods and if they pile up in your digestive tract, you are risking unnecessary aches and constipation.

2) Carbohydrates in general tend to satisfy your appetite quickly, all too quickly. If they make you lose your appetite for the fat and protein you also need, they will throw the balance of your diet out of kilter and cause you considerable trouble.

3) If the extra carbohydrates are in the form of refined sugar, they will increase your chances of developing tooth decay.

So beware of overdoing carbohydrates. But beware of underdoing them too. You need the quick and convenient energy they provide for physical exercise. Your brain needs them—glucose is its only food. You need them to burn up the fat you eat. If you don't eat enough carbohydrates, your muscles will not be operating at full efficiency. It is true that the process of neoglycogenesis will create sugar out of fats and proteins if your intake of carbohydrates is too low, but this is making your organism do unnecessary and possibly fatiguing work. You are better off getting your sugar straight, in the form of carbohydrates.

Carbohydrates come for human consumption in three forms:

Starches, which are to be found in bread, grain products, potatoes, rice, tapicoa, dried beans and peas, etc.

Sugars, found in the form of pure sugar or in honey, candy, chocolate, jams and jellies, and as an important ingredient of fruits and green vegetables.

Cellulose, the woody tissue of plants, which the human

body (unlike that of cows and horses) is not equipped to absorb but which is necessary to provide bulk or roughage so that the digestive process can proceed at a normal rate. Up to a point, cellulose provides a gentle laxative effect and is thus good for you, but too much of it can irritate your intestines and also carries off valuable hydrogen and calcium in your feces. The main sources of cellulose are vegetables, fruits and grain products.

You can get the proper distribution of carbohydrates by eating 200 grams of bread (eight or nine slices) a day; 350 grams of potatoes (about three medium-sized) a day—replaced three or so times a week by rice or pasta, and once or twice a month by dried beans or peas; 100 grams of other grain products (mostly breakfast cereal, with some flour for an occasional piece of pastry); 45 grams of sugar (about three tablespoons); 45 grams of jam or honey. Translated into calories, this will come up to 55% of your day's total intake, when you add to it the carbohydrates you get from milk (which you take principally for its protein value) and from fruits and vegetables (which as we will see you take chiefly for their vitamins).

The chief difference between the two kinds of carbohydrates you can absorb—sugars and starches—is that the latter takes considerable time to digest while the former is transformed into energy almost immediately. That is why sugar remains an essential part of the athlete's or any other diet, despite all the bad things that have been said about it. At moments of high tension, the sugar content of your blood, on which you depend for energy, can fall precipitately, by as much as 70%. You need to replenish it quickly to stave off collapse, and the quickest and most efficient way of doing so is to ingest some raw sugar or honey.

The trouble with sugar is that the form in which it is almost always taken in the modern world—refined—is totally lacking in vitamin B_1. If too much of your daily ration is in the form of refined sugar, you won't be getting enough of this essential vitamin. Therefore, you must never let your daily sugar intake exceed 10% of the calories you absorb on any one day. Remember that this 10% does not include just the lumps of sugar you put in your coffee or tea. It also includes honey, chocolate, jam, jelly, Coca-Cola, desserts.

There are always fads and fashions in athletic nutrition, and at present there is one for stuffing competitors with carbohydrates for three or four days preceding the Event. The medical evidence is inconclusive: some investigators report considerably improved performance after the carbohydrate-stuffing, others report no difference at all. My own experience leads me to side with the latter. In general, I do not approve of sudden tinkering with a well-functioning organism. Leave well enough alone. The chances of causing digestive disturbances with all that extra carbohydrate seem to me to outweigh any hypothetical benefits that might come from it.

I believe that the sensational results sometimes shown by athletes who have been given special force-feeding diets comes from the fact that they were, very simply, not being fed properly before. No test that I am aware of has been conducted in enough depth to prove that the force-feeding is responsible for the improved performance, if any. I am of the opinion of a wise old French doctor who had seen and studied many of these wonder processes in his lifetime and who concluded: "The gain in energy comes rather from the reserves accumulated during the training period than from any pre-game debauch, which may well disturb all the metabolisms of the body."

Fats, proteins, and carbohydrates do not exhaust the list of your nutritional needs. To be alive and healthy you need other things, things which are not technically nutrients but which you cannot do without just the same.

WATER

Water provides you with no energy, but it is an absolutely vital element of your daily diet. Men have gone for weeks without solid food—I think one Indian fakir made it to 62 days—but no one has ever stayed healthy more than four or five days without water.

Most of your body, in fact, is composed of water. It gradually dries up as you grow older. As a newborn babe you were 85% water, when you are old you will be down to 60%. Hence the Chinese proverb: the older you get the more you need to laugh and drink.

A man normally excretes about three liters of water per day, a woman about two and a half. All this must be replaced in your daily diet. A good half of this daily intake is in solid food (a peach or an onion, for example, is 89% water, meat is between 50 and 65, even a roasted peanut is 2% water). The rest you have to drink—eight or nine big glasses a day, all taken between meals for best results. (You may subtract a glass for every three cups of tea or coffee you drink.) Most people tend to drink too little water, and thus they put undue strain on their kidneys and bladder.

All recent studies emphasize the importance of water to the body at the time of sustained physical effort. This effort creates surpluses of pyruvic and lactic acids in the blood, which lead to fatigue. The more water you drink the more efficiently you can clean the acids out.

The more effort you exert, the more water you need: one cubic centimeter of water for every calorie. If you are in heavy training and need 3,500 or 4,000 calories a day, you should increase your water ration to three and a half or four liters respectively.

MINERALS

A number of minerals are necessary in your daily diet, some of them only in tiny quantities. A well-balanced diet will provide you automatically with virtually all that you need.

Sodium

A few pinches of the ordinary table salt we put on our food provide more sodium than is needed under most conditions. Most people oversalt their food, which generally contains some sodium itself and does not really need to be supplemented. But an athlete under extreme strain, or performing in hot weather, may need extra salt. Sodium presents the advantage of having an attraction for water, it helps keep it in your tissues when you need it for your effort, instead of pouring out prematurely in sweat. Two to five grams of salt tablets, depending on the degree of heat, can help out when taken before or during activity.

Potassium

You need potassium to enable your muscles to contract. If your supply runs low, you will get bad cramps. Anyone who eats fruits and vegetables and drinks milk in the course of the day will more than meet his need for potassium. But as in the case of sodium, you may need a small supplement at moments of great effort or great heat—from one half to three grams of gluconate of potassium taken before or during activity.

Chlorine

A pinch of table salt covers all your daily requirements.

Phosphorus

Phosphorus is necessary for the combustion that releases energy in your muscles and your brain. Athletes need more than ordinary people, but a well-balanced diet provides more than enough, except for very long and intense efforts, when a supplement should be taken in the form of tricalcic phosphate. I will talk of such exceptional circumstances later, when discussing individual sports.

You will find phosphorus in meat, fish, eggs, grain products, milk; it is hard to miss.

Sulphur

Sulphur helps rid the body of toxins, particularly the toxins of fatigue. Almost all protein products contain it, but it is most concentrated in dried beans, peas, lentils, etc. These should form a staple of your diet, but since they tend to be indigestible, I recommend taking them only once or twice a month, which is ample for your needs.

Iodine

If you don't get enough iodine, you will develop a goiter. In the not too distant past whole regions were afflicted with this unsightly condition, but the wide use of iodized salt has made it an anachronism.

Magnesium

Lack of magnesium can lead to lack of energy and extreme fatigue. Recent research indicates that the average modern diet is somewhat deficient in magnesium. You can get all you need by eating whole-wheat bread, chocolate and green vegetables, but large quantities of bread and chocolate can be hard on your digestion, so your doctor may advise taking three grams of lactate of magnesium daily instead.

Trace minerals

These include fluorine, zinc, cobalt, nickel, lithium, barium, arsenic, manganese. Nutritionists generally assume they are all necessary to human life, though no one knows exactly why because they occur so generally and in such small quantities that it is impossible to isolate them and conduct experiments to study their effects. The important thing for you to know is that they are all present in apparently adequate quantities in a well-rounded daily diet.

Calcium

Calcium is essential for your bones and teeth. Rickets in children, bone decay in adults, tooth trouble in both result from lack of it. It is also necessary for muscular contraction, and a shortage of calcium will lead to cramps.

The only adequate source of calcium is milk and milk products, and you can never afford to skimp on these in your diet.

Whole grains, chocolate, and some vegetables like spinach, chard, and rhubarb work against the body's absorption of calcium. It is most unlikely, however, that you will eat the considerable quantities that would be required to do you any serious harm. And if you do, you need only drink more milk, or eat more citrus fruits, which stimulate the body's absorption of calcium. Once again, a balanced diet helps even things out.

Iron

Iron provides the hemoglobin of the red blood corpuscles, and if you run short of it you will not have enough oxygen carried to where it is needed in your body. The consequences can be grave.

You do not need much, about 15 mg. a day, less than can be found in one slice of liver or one chocolate bar.

Meat in general is high in iron, and milk is low.

Copper

Copper, like iron, is needed in small quantities, which can be found more than adequately in meat but is lacking in milk.

A last word on minerals: it is important to keep a balance between calcium-rich products (milk, fruit and vegetables) and phosphorus-rich products (meat, grain products). This is because the former leave an alkaline residue in the body after digestion, the latter an acid one. You don't want your body to swing to either extreme. An imbalance in favor of phosphorus may force your body to dig into its own calcium reserves, leading to a weakening of bones and teeth. To keep an ideal balance, the ratio between calcium and phosphorus should be about two:-three. A well-balanced diet like the one I am going to spell out for you in the next chapter takes care of this automatically.

VITAMINS

Vitamins have been compared to precision workers overlooking the incredibly complex steps of the processes by which proteins, fats, and carbohydrates are broken down and put to use by your body. It is pleasant to know that if you eat wisely, as your omniverous tastes suggest—in other words if you follow a balanced diet—you will be taking in almost exactly the proper amount of vitamins for the work they have to perform.

This was illustrated for medical researchers on a nationwide scale in German-occupied France between 1940 and 1944. Undernourishment was almost universal and often severe. But there were almost no cases of specific vitamin-deficiency diseases like pellagra which comes from a lack of vitamin B_3, or PP. This was because the severely rationed food that was available, though insufficient for good health in general, was fairly well balanced. There was never enough meat, or milk, or vegetables, or bread, but the proportions between them happened to be approximately correct. The result was that the body received just about the amount of vitamins it needed to handle the food it was getting. After the war, rationing was ended and people were free to make up their own menus again. Many of them began overloading on items they had missed most during the period of restriction, especially bread. They got very fat and began showing all the symptoms of B_1 deficiency, constant fatigue and difficulty of movement.

There are by present count some 40 vitamins at work in our bodies, and there are probably more yet to be discovered.

They are all necessary for the proper functioning of the body, and if you go short in any one of them you will develop a deficiency state or disease which can hurt or even cripple you. Vitamin-deficiency diseases are almost always caused by defective diets. In modern times they are rarely due to poverty or the unavailability of proper foods; they are often the result of following fads which call for unbalancing the diet. Radical vegetarians, for instance, who eschew everything from the animal kingdom, including milk, run the risk of being seriously short of B_{12}.

A good balanced diet will take care of your vitamin needs under normal conditions. But you need supplemental doses of some vitamins under certain conditions of severe physical stress, and I will take these up in turn.

Vitamin B₁ (thiamine)

Thiamine, save my child! says the American poet Felicia Lamport, and indeed we would all of us be lost without it. B_1 is necessary for the metabolism of carbohydrates, it protects the nervous system, and it has a role to play in the sex glands. It is absolutely essential to have it, and have it in sufficient quantities in your daily food. Like all the so-called water-soluble vitamins, it cannot be stocked in your body, you have to get some in every day.

Fortunately, it is to be found in considerable quantities in many foods: meat (especially liver), green vegetables, whole-grain cereals. It is also found in yeast, and many people take yeast tablets to keep themselves high in B_1. But you should get plenty in your ordinary foods.

Some experimenters have given athletes massive doses of B_1 before sporting events to see if it improves their performance. Some report that it does, often in spectacular fashion. Others report that it has no effect at all. I suspect that the explanation, as in the case of most such discrepancies and contradictions in similar experiments, lies in the haphazard choice of subjects for the experiment: no one bothers to find out what their diet was before the extra doses began. My own feeling is that the athletes whose performance improved were short of B_1 to begin with. The ones whose performance did not improve had been eating properly; their bodies simply got rid of the extra B_1 and went on working adequately as they had before.

What would make athletes short of B_1? Well, they might have been drinking too much, and alcohol not only destroys vitamin B_1, but the lack of B_1 tends to increase the desire for alcohol.

Or they may have been following a diet over-heavy in

raw fish and shellfish, which contain a substance that tends to prevent the intestine from absorbing vitamin B_1. (The substance is destroyed by cooking.) This is highly unlikely: it would take prodigious quantities of raw fish or oysters to do any serious damage.

A much more likely cause is eating too much sugar. Refined sugar not only contains no vitamin B_1, but tends to take away your appetite for other foods which do contain it, and which you need all the more because your body needs sizeable quantities of B_1 to metabolize the sugar it ingests.

If for any reason you are short of vitamin B_1, a small dose (a 5- or 10-mg. pill), taken during the course of a meal once a day should suffice.

Vitamin B_6 or pyridoxine

This vitamin plays an important role in various metabolic processes involving carbohydrates, and fats, but especially proteins. It helps eliminate waste protein products, helps transport the amino acids that are used to create muscle tissue, and helps keep nerve tissue healthy. It is especially important when protein is being used as a source of energy, and athletes who for one reason or another are temporarily on a high-protein diet may need a supplementary dose of 15 to 30 mg. at the time of the Event. Under ordinary conditions and with a well-balanced diet, there is enough vitamin B_6 in your food to cover all your needs.

Vitamin B_{12} or cyanocobalamine

This highly beneficial vitamin, among its many other useful roles, facilitates the integration of amino acids into the body tissues. It is a vital factor in growth and in maintaining a steady weight.

It is found in animal products, especially in liver,

which is the organ which stocks it in the body. If you are not a vegetarian—and not anemic, in which case your doctor will undoubtedly recommend sizeable doses of B_{12}—you should be getting plenty of it in your daily diet. A single exception: if considerable muscle masses are involved (as in weight-lifting), a modest supplement of 150-200 mg. can help in the process of turning proteins into body tissue and removing toxins.

Vitamin C or ascorbic acid

This vitamin has a particularly strong influence on our general state of health and well-being. An ordinary person needs from 75 to 100 mg. a day, an active athlete twice as much.

Fortunately, it is found to some degree (often a high degree) in all fruits and vegetables, and since our diet calls for some of these at every meal, you should have no problem.

You should be aware of the fact, however, that a problem can arise owing to the relative fragility of this vitamin. The risk of its fading away is very high. The longer it takes a fruit or vegetable to get to you, the less vitamin C it is going to contain. Hence, if the fresh produce in your market comes from a long way off, you may be better off with a properly canned fruit or vegetable, where you can be sure the vitamin C has been sealed in at the cannery.

Beware of overdosing yourself with vitamin C. If you want to take it for a short time for therapeutic purposes, to fight off a cold for example, that is one thing. But taking substantial daily doses of more than 300 mg. over long periods of time can lead to many disturbances—diarrhea, cramps, insomnia. Even if it doesn't, the extra vitamins you swallow (and pay for) will do you no nutritional good whatever: the organism quickly gets rid of whatever it does not need.

I once had to treat a rugby player who was in a state of

total collapse; his adrenal glands had almost stopped functioning. It turned out that four years previously he had begun taking vitamin C pills because he was feeling weak. The more he took, the weaker he felt, and the more he kept stuffing down. He had reached the colossal total of three grams a day, when he found he couldn't stand up anymore. It took six months to get him back on his feet.

Vitamin B2 or riboflavin

This vitamin is important in various metabolic processes. It is found extensively in common foods, and no supplement should ordinarily be necessary. A therapeutic dose of up to 15 mg. may be found useful if you suffer from muscle cramps following severe activity.

Vitamin B3 or *PP;* nicotinic acid

It is found in meat and in grain products, and if you eat anything like a normal diet there is no danger of your getting pellagra, which is the disease caused by deficiency in B3. A well-balanced daily ration will amply cover the 20 mg. needed for a normal day's activities, or the 40 which the active athlete may require.

Vitamin B8 or *H;* biotin

The normal need is 5 mg. a day; an athlete may need 20 to 30. It is present in so many foods that the only way you could run short would be to restrict your diet almost entirely to egg whites, since they contain a substance which destroys it.

Vitamin B5 or pantothenic acid

This is found in so many foods, that a shortage is inconceivable. It plays a role in many vital bodily processes, including the Krebs cycle we discussed when following a piece of bread through your system.

Vitamin B9 or folic acid

This plays a part in the metabolism of certain amino-acids and nucleo-proteins.

It is found in the green leaves of vegetables like spinach, and also in animal kidneys and livers. A well-balanced daily diet will amply take care of your needs in this vitamin.

Fat-soluble vitamins

Unlike the water-soluble ones we have been discussing, these can be stocked in the fat in your body cells. There is no point, however, in swallowing a bottleful at intervals. A proper daily diet will ensure you a sufficient and regular intake.

The fat-soluble vitamins are A, D, E, and K.

Vitamin A

This is necessary for the proper functioning of your eyes, and for the proper growth and maintenance of your skin and mucous membrane. It is found in milk, butter, cod liver, and in the colored parts of fruit and vegetables.

A balanced diet contains all that you might conceivably need, unless you are practicing some sport at night or in darkness (automobile rallies, spelunking, etc.) or in dazzling light (cross-country skiing or mountain-climbing) in which case a daily supplement of 50,000 International Units is recommended.

Vitamin D

This is really a group of substances whose principal

role is to regulate the absorption of calcium and phosphorus in the intestines and direct them toward the bones and teeth. Its lack can lead to rickets in children, decalcification of the bones in adults. It also plays an important role in maintaining muscle tone.

The rays of the sun help activate the vitamin D we get from a variety of foods (cod-liver oil is the richest source). In these days, when milk is generally fortified with vitamin D, there is no danger of any deficiency, and there is no reason to take any supplement.

Vitamin E

This vitamin, necessary for reproduction, is adequately present in a normal diet and need not concern us here. Some American coaches in the 1950's thought that massive doses of vitamin E would make supermen out of ordinary athletes, but the days of that particular illusion appear to be over.

Vitamin K

This vitamin, which is necessary for your blood to be able to coagulate, is also found in ample quantities in the normal daily diet.

To sum up the subject of vitamins: a well-balanced diet should cover all your basic needs, except for the few cases noted above. If an examination shows that you are lacking in some vitamin or other, try balancing your diet according to the precepts of this book. If that doesn't work, you need further investigation by a doctor.

If during the stress and strain of arduous training and competition you find that you do need supplements, I would recommend taking multivitamin pills instead of large doses of individual vitamins. The composition of the pills is calculated to provide the right proportions and make sure that one vitamin doesn't work against another. It is all too easy to misjudge your own needs and end up by doing yourself more harm than good. It is conceivable that a heavy overdose of B₁ could actually cause pellagra by killing off all your supply of B₃. Too much vitamin A can block the absorption of vitamin C in the kidneys.

Gulping handfuls of miscellaneous vitamins every day may not necessarily hurt you. But the only people who are likely to profit by it are the stockholders in the drug companies.

Now, a last word about *hormones*. We are only at the threshold of understanding the complexity of the world of our hormones. The discovery that intense muscle activity causes a drain on our hormones is a fairly recent one.

Researchers have been all too quick to start experimenting with hormonal supplements in the way of doses or injections. I am convinced that all the extra nourishment your glands may need in time of effort can come from the ordinary food on your table. If an examination, for example, reveals that you are running short of thyroid in moments of stress, eat a few oysters.

The normal healthy human being has a hormonal production sufficient for his or her own use. Adding to it artificially can easily upset some delicate balance. Nutritionists above all others should avoid casting themselves in the role of sorcerer's apprentice.

IV
The Training Ration

We have now seen what you need, and how much, and why, to keep yourself properly fed so as to make the best possible use of your capacities.

I will now sum it all up in a simple daily diet which I call the Training Ration because I worked it out step by step with hundreds of athletes while they were actively and seriously preparing for competition. It is easy to follow, calls for no drugs or shots or exotic substances or practices; the foods it calls for can be found in anybody's larder or local supermarket.

As its name indicates, this diet was constructed for athletes in training, who wanted to get the very best out of their bodies. You don't have to be an athlete or even to be very active to get some benefit out of it. How closely you choose to follow the Training Ration depends both on your temperament and on how much importance you attach to the Event you are preparing for. If you are only looking forward to a friendly weekend game of golf, you don't have to follow my advice to the letter, only keep it in mind as an ideal which you should try to approximate, even when you are tempted to stray down the paths of self-indulgence. If, on the other hand, that weekend game involves your prestige, or a sizeable bet, you might find it advisable to follow this Training Diet religiously.

I have often been struck by how seemingly small changes in diet can have considerable effect. The finely tuned engine of an athlete's body can respond to quite minute modifications of the quantity and quality of its fuel—a good reason for never changing either too abruptly or too radically. When I was first consulted by Jean-Claude Killy, he was already a great skier, but his performances were uneven; he would be superb one week and only excellent the next. Part of the trouble was that he was still suffering the after-effects of a hepatitis he had picked up while serving in the French army in Algeria, and this could be taken care of by proper treatment. But another part was dietary—he was eating and drinking a bit too much. I had him cut down from one-half to one-quarter bottle of wine a day, and reduce his fat intake by a few grams. The violent variations in his performance from week to week disappeared.

The Training Ration which worked so well for Killy and the other athletes I have studied should work equally well for you. Even though the exact amount of food you take in depends on your own build and personal characteristics, the proportions of the various foods will be the same for whatever your size, condition, or the nature of the event you are preparing for. Whether you are bulky or slim, whether you have a hearty appetite or a finicky one, whether you are in training for a 100-yard dash or for climbing Mount Everest or just for a jog around Central Park, the basic rules, ingredients, and proportions remain the same.

At the moment of performance, when the long days of training are over and the Event is finally at hand, you may be faced with different dietary necessities and choices. It stands to reason that you won't be able to eat anything during a 100-yard dash while you would have to eat a good deal on your way up and down Everest. We will discuss this problem in detail a couple of chapters later. But such differences apply only to the actual day or days on which the Event takes place. During all the period when you are preparing for it, the Training Ration is identical for all.

Let me sum up the basic proportions as they were worked out in the last chapter. Your daily diet should consist of the following, and only the following:

- 15% of your daily caloric intake should be in the form of proteins. Assuming a daily total of 3,200 (2,700 for women), this comes to about 480 (405) calories of proteins to be distributed through your day's meals. More than half of them should be of animal origin.
- 30% should be in the form of fats, making some 960 (810) calories.
- 55% of carbohydrates, making some 1,760 (1,630) calories, of which a maximum of 10% should be provided by refined sugar (this includes honey, syrups, candy, etc.). If you take any alcoholic drinks, their calories should come to no more than 4% of your day's ration, i.e., 128 (108), to be subtracted from your carbohydrate quota.
- Plus a minimum of one to one and a half liters of water.

Except in some special circumstances which will be mentioned later, this is largely sufficient for your needs in every form of nutrition, including vitamins and mineral salts; and no supplements of any kind are needed.

The 15-30-55 proportions remain the basic law. I would also like to lay down a few by-laws of alimentary hygiene which I urge you to follow as they can save you much grief and inconvenience:

1) Eat slowly. Chew your food as much as you can before you swallow it. Hard crackers and biscuits or toast are better for you than soft bread. People who bolt their food (I am one of them, so I know whereof I speak) are depriving themselves of the services of two important agents, one mechanical and the other chemical, which your body conveniently provides to make it easier for you to absorb your food. One is your teeth, the other is your saliva. When food stays in your mouth for a while, you break it up with your teeth, and the salivary juices start working on the long process of decomposition we followed in the last chapter. The more work your salivary glands can do, the less time and effort your stomach will have to expend on the food, and the whole digestive process will go more quickly and smoothly. This is especially important if you are eating before any physical effort. You don't want solid chunks of food in your stomach taking up needless attention at a time when your body should be concentrating on other things.

2) Make sure that your food looks good as well as tastes good. Try to eat in surroundings that are pleasant rather than depressing. This is not always easy if the choice of your menu and place of eating is set by some impersonal authority. But do your best; remember that if you honestly enjoy a meal, it is better nourishment for both body and brain than the same amount of calories served tastelessly in disagreeable surroundings. This is because unpleasant sensations at the moment of eating disrupt the delicate contacts between your brain and your digestive organs. The brain doesn't send its signals through the nerves as regularly or as accurately as it should, your pyloric valve doesn't open at the proper moments, and food either goes into your intestines too soon or stays in your stomach too long and produces reactions of distress in either case.

3) By the same token, vary your food as much as possible. As you will see, my Training Ration allows you considerable leeway at every meal; in fact, there is no single

item on it which cannot be replaced by one or more sub-stitutes. You should make a deliberate effort to look for substitutes often. Monotony dulls the appetite, and I have seen all too many athletes and schoolchildren turn to sweet soda pop and other abominations not so much be-cause they liked the stuff as because they were bored to death by the theoretically nutritious but hopelessly unin-teresting institutional meals they were being subjected to every day. You need a full day's ration every day, and you will get more cooperation from your appetite by keeping the ration interesting.

4) Do not drink during meals. Putting liquid in your mouth at the same time as food dilutes your salivary juices and makes them work less efficiently, just as if you ate too fast. And when it goes down into your stomach, it dilutes your gastric juices too, and interferes correspond-ingly with their work.

5) I believe it was Thomas Jefferson who said that one should always get up from the table feeling a little bit hungry, and his rule remains a good one for all to follow. Overeating will give you a stuffed, drowsy feeling that cannot help but lower your efficiency in whatever you may be doing.

6) Remember that your own body is your own best guide, and you should give it every chance to tell you what it really likes and doesn't like. Unfortunately, many of us are all too willing to pick up odd and irrational prej-udices and then ascribe them to our own experience. Many people will tell you, for example, that eggs are indi-gestible because eggs repeat on them. As a matter of fact, eggs are easily digestible for the great majority of peo-ple—what causes the trouble is generally the grease in which they have been cooked. Try a fresh three-minute egg someday, and see if it is really hard to digest. It may, of course, be that you are one of the small minority whose bodies really can't stand eggs, and in that case it would be folly to keep forcing them down. There are plenty of other

sources of good animal protein available, and room for the most catholic not to say eccentric tastes. If like the witches in *Macbeth* you enjoy putting the eyes of newts and toes of frogs in your stewpot, I have no nutritional objection, so long as you keep in good shape and your weight doesn't start yawing alarmingly up and down.

7) Try to arrange to spread your food intake evenly through the day. Do not bunch up a majority of your daily calories at any one meal.

Be sure especially to have a substantial breakfast. My own and some other European peoples have the very bad habit of skipping breakfast almost entirely. They have nothing but a cup of black coffee, sometimes with a lethal shot of applejack in it, into which they may dunk a piece of bread. Such a meal, or pseudo-meal, represents a whole collection of nutritional sins in concentrated form: there is no nourishment to speak of, since there are no calories in the coffee; the alcohol on an empty stomach is many times more dangerous than on a full one; and the soggy bread is swallowed without being chewed and puts an unnecessary burden on the stomach. Taking a breakfast like this means in effect that you are starving yourself for 16 hours, or two-thirds of the day, between last night's dinner and today's lunch, and no matter how much you ate at dinner it cannot carry you in condition through all that stretch. No wonder that statistics in a number of French and Belgian towns have indicated a sudden rise in the number of automobile accidents around noon. After 16 hours of fasting, the drivers are bound to be jumpier, their reflexes are less dependable than they would be if they had eaten intelligently. Not to speak of the fact that they may have put an aperitif or two on an empty stomach, compounding all their sins and making them even more accident-prone than before.

Bearing all these bits of wisdom in mind, we can now turn to the construction of our basic Training Ration, with brief notes showing just why each item has its place in it.

Breakfast

• One bowl of cereal with milk and sugar. This gives you a good supply of energy-rich carbohydrates to start the day. Since the same kind of cereal can become boring, vary it as much as possible, but stick to simple types like cornflakes or oatmeal, avoiding at all costs the fancy over-sugared brands. You can vary the menu still more by replacing the cereal every few days by a slice of lean ham or some lean bacon or cold cuts (or one egg and half a slice of meat); in this case you should replace one of the meat dishes in a later meal by a starchy product like rice or potatoes.

• One slice of toast with butter or margarine, and one with jam or honey. This will give you some good and easily digestible carbohydrates, with a little fat for balance. Your muscles will be getting two kinds of energy-supplying sugar here; the sugar in the jam or honey will go directly to your muscles, while the starch of the toast will take longer to process into sugar and will feed out energy to you later in the course of the morning.

• A glass of orange juice or half a grapefruit or any other fruit (make sure it is ripe, or you may get diarrhea) or a glass of tomato juice. This will provide you with vitamin C, as well as a little more sugar for energy.

• One cup of tea or coffee, with up to three lumps of sugar. The caffeine which is found in both of these beverages is a tonic which can help you wake up. In addition, a hot drink is advisable in the morning to help clear your upper digestive tract of any left-overs, bits of digestive debris that have piled up in it overnight. On the other hand caffeine (which has no nutritive value) can make you nervous, so if you would rather avoid it, you may replace the tea or coffee with a cup of vegetable broth. One way or the other, you will be helping along your daily intake of liquids. Remember not to put cream in your coffee or tea; the cholorogenic acid in the coffee will mix with the albumen in the cream to form lumps in your stomach. If you don't like it sweet, don't sugar it but take more honey with your toast and a little more fruit juice.

Midday meal

• One vegetable salad. The vegetable can be either raw (lettuce, celery, carrots, tomatoes) or cooked (beets), with a dressing of lemon juice and oil. This dish provides you with a good deal of water, mineral salts, vitamins, and enough cellulose to give some bulk without irritating your intestines. Taken at the start of the meal, it stimulates your reflexes of gastric secretion and will help you digest the rest of your meal better.

• One serving of roast or broiled or boiled meat or fish with no sauce or gravy. This provides protein both to repair the wear and tear on your muscle tissues since the previous day and to build up new tissue as well.

• One cooked green vegetable, or one starchy food (potatoes, rice, pasta). But not both at once: the one you don't have at lunch should be on your menu in the evening. They can be served with a little melted butter or margarine. The starchy foods will provide you with considerable energy. The green vegetables, though they are generally regarded as being exceptionally nutritious, do not really have very much to offer you. They are rich in water and contain mineral salts, but you can easily get all you need of these from other sources. Their vitamins are generally lost in the cooking process; they do provide some bulk, which helps prevent constipation. But their chief advantage is a negative one: since you have to eat something to fill your stomach, they take up space which you might otherwise be tempted to fill with undesirable amounts of other foods like sweets.

• One or two pieces of toast.

- Cheese or yogurt. This provides you with calcium and mineral salts in addition to protein.
- A ripe fruit, a good source of the vitamin C which you have to keep taking more or less constantly.

Afternoon snack
- A cup of tea, or a glass of milk.
- Biscuits or crackers or toast with butter, margarine or jam.

This light snack helps spread your food intake through the day, so that too much of it won't pile up at a single meal.

Evening meal
- One bowl of vegetable soup with tapioca or vermicelli or noodles. You can have vegetables in the soup or not as you wish; what is important is the liquid into which most of the good of the vegetables has passed, and which will serve as a vehicle for eliminating toxins that have piled up in your liver and kidneys.
- One serving of meat, fish or (occasionally) eggs. Another helping of proteins to provide you with the essential amino acids your body needs.
- One serving of cooked green vegetables, or starchy food (whichever you didn't have for lunch), served with melted butter or margarine.
- One piece of cheese or a glass of milk.
- One ripe fruit, or a dish of stewed or canned fruit, or a piece of light pastry.

Any of these elements can be switched about from meal to meal as you like. It is best, however, to space your food more or less evenly among your three main meals.

I have deliberately not given the size of portions or servings above because you have to work them out for yourself in consideration of your special needs. Assuming a daily need of 3,200 calories, your daily totals in each of the principal categories would be about as follows: (If you need more or less, adjust them accordingly; be sure to adjust them *all* accordingly.)

A. Carbohydrates
- Two hundred grams of bread (eight or nine slices).
- Three hundred and fifty grams of potatoes (three medium-sized). This should be your basic starch. Replace it two or three times a week by rice or spaghetti or some other form of pasta. And once or twice a month replace it by dried beans or peas, either mashed or in a soup. They are not easy to digest, which is why it is best not to eat them too often, but they are particularly rich in sulphur, which helps you eliminate toxins.
- One hundred grams of grain products, in the form of breakfast cereal and occasionally pastry.
- Forty-five grams of sugar.
- Forty-five grams of honey or jam.

B. Proteins
- Two hundred and fifty grams of meat. The meat can be replaced two or three times a week, or more often if you wish, by fish; and once a week it should take the form of liver.
- Four to five eggs in the course of a week.
- Three-quarters of a pint of milk a day.
- Fifty grams of cheese.

These last two items, the milk and cheese, should be doubled in the ration of adolescents who need the extra calcium. But they don't need extra fat, so they should be sure to take this supplement in the form of fat-free milk or cheese.

If for one reason or another you don't want meat at a meal, note that half a liter of milk or two eggs give the protein equivalent of 100 grams of meat. As already noted, milk can be substituted for meat at any time, but meat cannot be substituted for milk; some form of milk product—cheese, yogurt or custard if you cannot support milk itself—is essential.

C. Fats
• Thirty grams—about two level (and make sure they are level) tablespoons of butter.
• Thirty grams of vegetable oil.
• Fifteen grams of vegetable shortening.

D. Water
• A liter and a half. This is quite a lot of water, especially to take between meals, as you should, and one of the most common nutritional sins is to forget to drink a full complement of water every day.

E. Alcohol
• Preferably none at all.
There has been considerable debate about the nutritional value of alcoholic beverages. Without getting involved in technicalities, let me say that such values are not completely non-existent, but they are outweighed very heavily and in very short order by the defects that go with them. We all know successful athletes who drink heavily, but I am sure they would be even more successful athletes if they did not. If you are willing to scale down your ambitions for the sake of the pleasures of a few extra drinks, that is your choice. But if you want the machine of your body to run at its topmost level, you will have to cut down your alcoholic intake to very modest proportions, if not suppress it entirely.

There is a long list of misdemeanors to be charged to alcohol. The momentary feeling of warmth that drinks can give you are soon, all too soon, replaced by depression and chill. Alcohol saps your vitamin reserves. It disturbs your reflexes and distorts your judgment, and I need not tell you that in large quantities it can cause serious and permanent damage to your nerves and your liver, both of

101

which are very hardy types of organs but which, once deteriorated, cannot be replaced.

Nevertheless, if—and only if—you are one of the happy few who can take a few drinks without being driven inevitably on to have many drinks, I find that a small daily absorption of alcohol does no particular harm, even to an athlete in heavy training, and if it makes you feel better, go right ahead. But be sure that you can stop, without any regrets at the absolute limit, which is 4% of your daily caloric intake. This works out to amounts which will seem small if not derisory to a serious drinker—about two glasses of table wine, or four of beer, or a couple of shots of whisky, gin or vodka. My personal preference, based only partly on national prejudice, is for the wine. Taken with some cheese at the end of your lunch or dinner, it may actually help the digestive process, by modifying the physical characteristics of proteins you have eaten, making them easier to digest. Beer has more nourishment than wine, in protein as well as carbohydrate form, but it presents the difficulty of being carbonated, which can start you burping when you should be paying attention to other things. A single shot of whisky is theoretically permissible at each meal, but few people I know are satisfied with a single shot of whisky.

I have talked quite confidently so far about exact proportions—15-30-55—and specific caloric values for the different dishes in your daily menu. I realize that this is not wholly realistic. Unless you have a full-time specialist buying, weighing and preparing your food, how in the world are you going to keep figures precise to the gram or calorie? Few of us can afford such a service, or would like it if we could get it. We live in a world where sometimes we scrape together our own meals, sometimes take potluck in the houses of friends, sometimes eat at training tables or in mess halls, sometimes we go to restaurants, or buy a sandwich at the ball park. How can we possibly know the exact weight, the exact ingredients, the exact caloric value of everything that passes our lips?

The best that can be hoped for, practically speaking, is a rough idea. It would be futile to ask for more. If you have to worry about the precise value of everything you see in front of you, you will only be losing precious energy.

If you follow the Training Diet I have just spelled out, you will be reasonably close to getting everything you need in the right doses. For that matter, if you follow the simplified 1-2-4 diet described in Chapter II, you will not be far off.

If you want to be more exact, the next chapter lists common foods in portions you might expect to find, with the number of calories you derive from each in the form of proteins, fats and carbohydrates. You can use it to analyze your food for a day or a week, and determine how close you are coming to the 15-30-55 ideal. You need not do this too often; unless you get a positive enjoyment out of playing with such figures, it would only get you involved in the kind of finicky calorie-counting which gives dieting a bad name. The important thing is to be thinking in terms of proportions, and the table may help you to do that. As time goes on, you will find you can judge the proportions of any given dish or meal more or less automatically, and judge at a glance if it is anywhere near the ideal.

How long should you follow this Training Diet? That is entirely up to you. There may be times when any diet at all is a strain and should be avoided. There are, after all, other things in life besides physical fitness, and people who think of nothing else are missing a good deal. But as long as physical fitness is a primary goal, and as long as you are in active and serious training for the Event which is going to engage all your powers of body and mind, you should make an effort to follow this Training Diet closely if not religiously.

And you should follow it right up to the day of the Event. I know the nervous strain gets pretty strong as the day approaches, and by the evening before the Event itself it may get very intense indeed. Many doctors as well as laymen have been tempted to tinker with their diets at this point. Some recommend eating more, some recommend eating less, some recommend eating nothing at all. Some want to stuff you up with meat, others with sugar. It is perfectly possible for one or another of these methods to give satisfactory results in individual cases, but I believe that on the whole they are not worth the effort: any sudden tinkering with the diet your body has gotten used to is likely to disorient it and cause trouble more serious than the worry and fretfulness it was supposed to prevent. A good, well-balanced diet is good for your whole body, including your nerves. And your nerves will be better able to support the strain of those last hours of waiting if you keep following the Training Ration right up to the day of the Event.

On that day the nature of the activity itself will force a change in your eating pattern, as we will discuss at length in a later chapter.

But meanwhile stick to the simple, wholesome, appetite-satisfying 15-30-55 standard. As long as there is nothing unusual about you that calls for special medical attention, and as long as you are keeping yourself in shape by regular exercise, you will be bound to feel better all along the line. Perhaps you won't even notice that you have stopped worrying about your weight anymore.

V
A Dictionary of Foods
for Fitness

In this chapter you will find an alphabetical list of most of the foods you are likely to see on your table, with remarks on their role and value in a diet aimed at maximum physical fitness.

I have classified these foods by a system borrowed from the one the famous Michelin Guide uses to judge the quality of restaurants.

Three stars (***), the highest category, is for food of high nutritional value that you can eat every day. *Can* eat, not *must* eat. There is no single item which is absolutely indispensable. But these three-star foods as a whole— milk, beef, fish, butter, vegetable oil, certain vegetables and fruits, bread and its starchy replacements (potatoes, rice, etc.)—should remain the basic elements of your diet. They are the joists and beams of your house of good health.

Two stars (**) indicates food which you should take regularly, but not every day: liver, for instance, which is an immensely valuable food but which would burden your system if you ate it much more than once a week.

One star (*) indicates foods which may or may not be good for you, depending on your personal make-up or personal tastes. If they agree with you, you may eat them as often as you want. If you find that something like cabbage is hard to digest, or something like strawberries makes you break out all over, you can leave them alone with an easy conscience.

No star at all means that this is a particular food which I cannot recommend for a diet aimed at physical fitness. This doesn't mean you have to abandon such foods forever. Alcohol, for instance, cannot possibly help you get into good shape, though a couple of glasses of wine a day will do you no harm. I do not expect, however, that you are going to restrict yourself to two glasses of wine a day for the rest of your life. Someday, even when you are in training, you may not be satisfied with two glasses, you may want to go on a toot, say to hell with everything. That is perfectly human, and there is nothing wrong with it if you have the willpower to stop your toot in time and get back to seriously taking care of yourself. As I have said before, there are no forbidden fruits in my diet. If you keep your eyes fixed on your goal of topnotch physical fitness, you will find it easier to keep your excursions in dangerous byways to a minimum.

Alongside each item of food, you will find three figures giving caloric counts—not the total for the food as a whole, which is of little interest and can be misleading, but the totals appearing in the form of proteins, fats, carbohydrates. You will thus get a much clearer idea of what you are actually taking in as nourishment. You do not need to memorize these figures, and you don't need to spend any more time with them than you feel like. If they help you to think of your food in terms of proportions, they will have more than served their purpose.

The figures refer to portions which the U.S. Department

of Agriculture, from whose excellent publications the tables are derived, regards as average. Of course it is unlikely that you will eat precisely these average portions. Your egg at breakfast may weigh more than the 50 grams of the Department of Agriculture's, and your portion of chicken need not be limited to three and a half ounces. You cannot expect perfect accuracy in these matters. But the figures given here are in practical enough form so that you should be able to use them as the basis for a reasonably accurate count. On any specimen day you can mark down on a piece of paper at each meal roughly how many calories of the three categories you have taken in. Add them up at the end of the day, and you can see how close you have come to the 15-30-55 balance which represents your ideal.

Trace (Tr) is an insignificant amount which you need not count. One cup equals one-half pound; eight ounces equal 16 tablespoons; one tablespoon equals three teaspoons; 100 grams equal three and a half ounces.

TABLE OF FOODS

*Almonds

P	F	C	
104	693	112	calories per cup.
6	43	7	calories per tablespoon.

Almonds provide a good source of essential fatty acids and of vitamin B_1. They are also rich in potassium. Their very high fat content makes it advisable to use them with discretion under ordinary circumstances: it is all too easy to pick up a few here and there and forget to count them in your daily fat ration, with disastrous consequences for your figure. But they can be invaluable when you have to carry with you a good source of energy concentrated into a small volume, as in mountain-climbing.

***Apples

P	F	C	
Tr	Tr	72	calories per apple.
Tr	Tr	120	calories per cup of apple juice.
4	Tr	244	calories per cup of sweetened apple-sauce.
4	Tr	104	calories per cup of unsweetened, or artificially sweetened, applesauce.

In addition to all their other well-known good qualities, apples contain pectin, which can help you economize on dental bills: an apple eaten at bedtime will help to dissolve cavity-causing sugar that has gotten lodged between your teeth.

***Apricots

P	F	C	
4	Tr	56	calories per 3 apricots.
20	9	248	calories per cup, cooked, unsweetened.
32	9	400	calories per cup dried (40 halves).

*Artichokes

P	F	C	
6	Tr	20	calories per artichoke.

An excellent food, but since it can cause flatulence, watch out for it when you are preparing any physical effort.

*Asparagus

P	F	C	
4	Tr	8	calories per 4 spears, cooked.

Go easy on asparagus; it contains a substance which can irritate the urinary canal and even bring on cystitis.

*Avocadoes

P	F	C	
20	333	52	calories per 10-ounce California avocado.

A very nourishing food, but also very high in fat content, as you can see from the accompanying figures. Take it easy if you have a weight problem.

***Bacon

P	F	C
20	72	4

calories per 2 slices (20 slices to the pound). So far as possible, eat only the lean. Cook it crisp.

*Bananas

P	F	C
4	Tr	104

calories per banana.

It is very easy to eat too many bananas, and that will make you fat. Besides, they are high in cellulose, which can irritate your intestines.

**Beans, dried

P	F	C
56	9	152
56	9	196

calories per cup of white beans.
calories per cup of lima beans.

With their high carbohydrate content these provide a good energy source. They also supply proteins, vitamins of the B group, and minerals, particularly iron and sulphur.

Unfortunately, they are also high in cellulose, and take quite a long time to digest. They should figure in your diet, but not more than once or twice a month. Mash them well to make digestion easier.

***Beans, green (or wax or yellow)

P	F	C
8	Tr	28

calories per cup, cooked.

Highly recommended at all times, provided they are young and fresh. Be sure not to overcook them, as their vitamins B1 and C and their mineral salts will be boiled away into the water. They should be cooked whole; cutting them into fine strips increases the surface through which these essential ingredients can escape.

***Beef

P	F	C	
129	69	0	calories per 100 grams (3½ ounces) of sirloin steak, broiled, trimmed of fat.
113	120	0	calories per 100 grams of rib roast, trimmed of fat.
120	85	0	calories per 100 grams of pot roast (trimmed of fat).
110	100	0	calories per 100 grams of hamburger, lean.
106	72	0	calories per 100 grams of corned beef, canned, lean.

Beef is an excellent source of proteins, rich in essential amino acids in a mixture well suited to the human organism. It is also rich in phosphorus, iron and vitamin B.

It is one of the hardest foods to measure accurately in terms of calories, for it is impossible to say how much fat there is in any given cut, or how much will run out during the cooking. The more expensive it is, the more fat it is likely to contain.

Common belief to the contrary, there is no nutritional difference whatever between rare (or raw) meat and well done.

Beef should always be started cooking at high heat, to seal in the nutritional values. The only ways to consider cooking it are these:

• Broiled or grilled. You don't use fat in this process, and some of the fat in the meat can run off.

• Panbroiled in a Teflon pan.

• Roasted. (The oven should be preheated for 15 minutes before putting the meat in.)

• Braised. A pot roast is a good way to cook inexpensive cuts of beef. Brown the meat in a very small quantity of hot shortening, then add potatoes, carrots or other vegetables and a little liquid, and cook slowly until tender.

• Boiled. The meat should be put into boiling salted water and simmered until tender. If you start cooking the meat in cold water, the nutritive elements will seep out into the liquid while it is heating. You may get a delicious soup (see *Soups*) but it won't be good for you, and the meat will be tasteless when done.

Hamburger has a great advantage over unchopped meat—particularly when the Event is looming—in that it takes less time to digest and therefore you run less risk of clogging up your system at a moment of crisis. But chopped meat is quick to spoil, so make sure that what you get is freshly ground. The best way to make sure is to grind it yourself.

***Beets

P	F	C	
4	Tr	28	calories per 100 grams (2 beets).

Make sure your beets are young and tender, not big and coarse and woody, which would scratch your intestinal lining.

If you are scared by seeing your urine turn blood-red, check back to see if you have eaten beets in the previous 24 hours before you run to a doctor.

Beverages, alcoholic

P	F	C	
0 (plus 100 for the alcohol)	0	Tr	calories per jigger (1½ ounces) of gin, rum, vodka, or whisky, 80 proof.
Tr (plus 69 from alcohol)	0	16	calories per glass (3½ ounces) of table wine.
4 (plus 90 from alcohol)	0	56	calories per 12-ounce glass of beer. (These figures are for domestic draught beer. Bottled and imported beers are apt to be higher in both carbohydrate and alcohol.)

Alcohol is absorbed immediately into the bloodstream, and, as every drinker knows, its immediate effect is apt to be a feeling of strength and energy, if not euphoria. This is, alas, accompanied by a diminution of the critical faculty and a slowing down of reflexes. Whatever benefit you get from alcohol comes out of the first swallow or so; from then on the net consequences are bound to be less than ideal from the standpoint of athletic or other performance.

It is not true that alcohol warms you up. You may certainly think it does, for your face flushes and your skin tingles. But this is a superficial phenomenon. The blood vessels at the surface of your body dilate, as they do when you make any muscular exertion, and you actually lose body heat in the process; it escapes through the skin while you are feeling that rosy glow. So do not put your trust in those friendly St. Bernards with the jug around their neck: it is possible they have killed as many travelers in the Alpine passes as they have saved.

If you want to go into serious training for any kind of Event, you will have to cut down on your alcoholic intake drastically. Preferably to zero, but at all events to no more than 4% of your total daily caloric intake. The best way to take it, in my opinion, is in the form of a couple of glasses of light red wine which, taken with a piece of cheese at the end of your meals, can actually help your digestion. Two shots of whisky or four glasses of beer would provide the same amount of alcohol, but I do not think they would help your digestion any.

Beer has some solid nutritional properties, but they are outweighed in my opinion by its drawbacks. One of these is its carbonization, which is bound to produce gas in your stomach, and should be strongly avoided before or during any form of physical activity.

You can see the effects of overindulgence in beer on any German or Scandinavian street; it is a terribly fattening drink. It also has another inconvenience which should give women drinkers pause. Beer is mostly barley, but depending on its strength and quality a certain amount of hops is generally used. Hops are extremely rich in estrogen, so rich that it seeps through the skin of

112

female workers in the hop fields, and no matter what stage of their cycle they are in when they start work, their periods begin within two days. Women who drink large quantities of hop-rich beer are playing dangerous games with their sexual hormones.

Beverages, carbonated

P	F	C	
0	0	148	calories per 12-ounce glass of cola.
0	0	116	calories per 12-ounce glass of ginger ale or quinine tonic.
0	0	0	calories per 12-ounce glass of artificially sweetened drinks.

You don't need gas in your stomach when you are preparing for physical effort. I would avoid these drinks.

***Blueberries

P	F	C	
4	9	84	calories per cup.

A good source of vitamin A.

***Bread

P	F	C	
8	9	52	calories per slice of white or rye bread (18 slices to a loaf).
12	9	48	calories per slice of whole wheat bread.
8	27	60	calories per 1 2-inch-diameter baking-powder biscuit.
12	36	80	calories per 1 corn muffin.
8	18	60	calories per 1 pan roll.
12	18	64	calories per 1 frankfurter or hamburger roll.
20	18	120	calories per 1 hard roll.

Most of the bread sold in stores is white bread made from wheat flour. It is rich in carbohydrates and therefore a good source of energy. It also has some protein, a good deal of phosphorus, and it generally comes enriched with vitamins.

There is no doubt in anyone's mind that bread is a necessary food; it has been called the staff of life for ages. But many people will tell you that ordinary store bread is deleterious to your health. I think they exaggerate.

It is true that the milling process which whitens the flour gets rid of a number of properties from the original grain, but nothing that you cannot replace from other sources. My chief quarrel with white store bread is not its whiteness but its softness. You tend to swallow it without chewing, and that deprives you of the valuable aid of your saliva in the digestive process. I recommend, therefore, toasting your bread, or eating hard biscuits, crackers, rusks, melba toast, anything that will call your teeth into action.

Whole wheat bread retains more of the original properties of the grain. These include its magnesium and also its cellulose (bran) which provides fiber you need to provide bulk in your intestines, but which may also make the bread more difficult to digest.

*Broccoli

P	F	C	
24	9	32	calories per 1 medium stalk.

Broccoli should be used with caution; it can cause gas and irritate your intestines.

*Brussels sprouts

P	F	C	
28	9	40	calories per cup (7 or 8 sprouts).

May be hard on tender intestines.

***Butter

P	F	C	
Tr	108	Tr	calories per tablespoon (1/8 of a 1/4-pound stick).
Tr	36	Tr	calories per 1-inch square pat.

Butter contains practically no protein or carbohydrate. It is basically composed of a little water and a lot of fat, unfortunately saturated fat which is not ideal for your body. But it also is our principal source of vitamin A and should figure in your diet every day. Sixty grams (about three tablespoons) is plenty.

Butter has a low burning point and will start to smoke at 120 degrees centigrade. Cooking it makes it lose most of its vitamins, but none of its cholesterol. It should therefore not be used for cooking foods, but be taken plain on bread, or melted on foods like vegetables or spaghetti or potatoes.

*Cabbage

P F C
8 Tr 16   calories per 1 cup, cooked.

Cabbage can be taken from time to time on your regular Training Diet, but should be avoided when the Event is coming up; it sometimes causes irritation of the colon.

It contains an amino acid which inhibits the produc-..on of thyroxin by the thyroid gland. Lack of thyroxin causes goiter, and there were actual cases of goiter reported among prisoners of war in Germany in World War II who had been kept on a diet consisting mostly of cabbage soup. Unless you restrict your own diet to cabbage soup, you have nothing to fear on this score.

Rumors have been spread that Russian athletes train and grow great on cabbage. But I have been informed by Soviet coaches at the Olympic Games that this is not so; they use cabbage only to make borscht, and sparingly at that.

*Cake, see pastry

*Candy

P F C
4 27 88   calories per 1 ounce of caramel.
4 36 84   calories per 1 ounce of fudge.
0 Tr 112 calories per 1 ounce of hard candy.

There is no reason why you can't take your daily sugar

ration under this form, so long as you remember that it *is* sugar and keep it within its proper limits.

*Cantaloupes

P   F   C
4   Tr   56   calories per ¹/₂ melon, 5 inches in diameter.

The cantaloupe is almost all water (91%) and has little nutritional interest. It is all right to take one occasionally, but beware: it is usually served chilled, and chilled food may cause your gall bladder to contract abruptly, flooding your digestive tract with bile and causing diarrhea. The French often start a meal with cantaloupe into which they pour a healthy slug of port wine. This warms up the fruit and solves the digestion problem, but adds others, since port wine on an empty stomach is a good way to get drunk.

***Carrots

P   F   C
4   Tr   20   calories per carrot (5¹/₂ inches long, 1 inch thick).

Carrots may be eaten raw or cooked. If raw, it is a good idea to grate them. Otherwise, you may get tired of chewing them and start swallowing with insufficient mastication.

The three-star rating I have given this vegetable applies only to young, tender carrots. As the vegetable ages, its cellulose gets tougher and can irritate your intestines.

Carrots contain (and give their name to) carotene, a hydrocarbon which not only gives them their attractive red color but turns to vitamin A in your body. You will need all the vitamin A you can get if you go in for sports like boxing which take place under artificial light. You will need it equally in places where there is not enough light, as in underground caves, or where there is too much, as in mountain snow. Carrots alone won't give you all the vitamin A you need—you would have to eat a bushel to get a really adequate source of supply.

*Cauliflower

P	F	C	
12	Tr	20	calories per 1 cup.

A member of the cabbage family, and the same observations apply.

*Caviar

P	F	C	
16	18	2	calories per 1 tablespoon.

Caviar has certain nutritional drawbacks (it is high in fat for one thing) and is also horribly expensive, but if you want to splurge on it once a year or so, why not?

***Celery

P	F	C	
Tr	Tr	8	calories per stalk.

See under *lettuce*.

***Cereals, breakfast

P	F	C	
8	Tr	84	calories per 1 cup cornflakes.
12	Tr	88	calories per 1 cup farina.
20	18	92	calories per 1 cup oatmeal.

Provided you don't eat the oversweetened kinds which are threatening to turn our children into a generation of sugar addicts, with big bellies and rumps and rotten teeth, cereals are an excellent way to start off a day's diet. The sugar you sprinkle on them gives you some quick energy, while the sugar you derive from their starch takes somewhat longer to reach your muscles and helps you keep going steadily through the morning.

***Cheese

P	F	C	
28	81	4	calories per 1 ounce American cheese.
28	81	4	calories per 1 wedge camembert type.
28	81	4	calories per 1 ounce cheddar.
24	81	4	calories per 1 ounce roquefort type.

P	F	C	
32	72	4	calories per 1 ounce Swiss.
4	54	Tr	calories per 1 cubic inch of cream cheese.
132	90	28	calories per 1 cup cottage cheese, creamed.
136	9	20	calories per 1 cup cottage cheese uncreamed.

Cheese has much the same nutritional properties as the milk from which it is made, except that it has less water, more fat, less calcium and somewhat less carbohydrate, which is changed into lactic acid during the fermentation process. The varying amount of fat in different types of cheese accounts for their wide range of caloric value. They are all rich in vitamins A, B_2 and B_{12}.

There is a common delusion that dry cheese, like Swiss and Parmesan, are "diet foods," which will help you lose weight. Not at all. The drier a cheese, the higher its fat content is likely to be.

If for one reason or another you don't like milk, cheese can always provide a satisfactory replacement.

***Cherries

P	F	C	
8	Tr	104	calories per cup.

*Chestnuts

P	F	C	
21	22	308	calories per cup.

Chestnuts are very rich in carbohydrates, hence in energy. They are also very rich in vitamins B_1 and C, and because of their thick skins they do not lose appreciable amounts of these vitamins in cooking, as so many other foods do.

Nevertheless, they are not easy to digest and should be eaten only on widely separated occasions.

***Chicken

P	F	C	
80	27	0	calories per 3-ounce serving.

Can be eaten at any meal where your diet calls for meat. Don't eat the skin.

**Chocolate

P	F	C	
8	81	64	calories per 1 ounce of milk chocolate.
4	70	48	calories per 1 ounce of semi-sweet.

Chocolate, with its high caloric content, is bursting with energy. It also has appreciable quantities of vitamins B and D; it satisfies the appetite easily and it possesses tonic and diuretic qualities. Unfortunately, its high fat content makes it hard to digest. And it contains calcium oxalate, which in large quantities is bad for your joints. It is best not to eat it regularly, and when you do, take it in small amounts. This does not apply to occasions when you are engaged in intense efforts like mountain-climbing or cross-country skiing, where chocolate provides an ideal energy-rich food concentrated into a small, easily portable volume.

***Citrus fruits

P	F	C	
4	3	64	calories per 1 orange.
8	4	104	calories per 1 cup of orange juice.
4	2	40	calories per 1 tangerine.
4	3	24	calories per 1 lemon.
2	2	112	calories per 1 cup diluted lemonade concentrate.
3	2	84	calories per 1 cup of lime juice.
4	2	48	calories per 1/2 grapefruit.
4	2	96	calories 1 per cup of grapefruit juice.

These are the highest of all foods in vitamin C, the vitamin of effort, and therefore indispensable in a healthy diet.

You may find it preferable to take them in the form of juice, since the cellulose of the pulp can be difficult to digest.

119

**Clams

P   F   C
22   5   4   calories per half-dozen clams.
See *oysters*

Coffee

P   F   C
Tr Tr Tr No calories to speak of per cup.

The essential ingredient of coffee, caffeine, has a stimulating effect on the nervous system which in small doses can facilitate physical and intellectual effort and fight off fatigue. But the average cup of coffee is not a small dose; it can contain 12 cg of caffeine.

Athletes tend to be jumpy enough as it is, and anybody is apt to be nervous on the eve of an Event. Drinking too much coffee at a time when you are already anxious can lead to considerable nervousness and bad insomnia.

I do not mean to insist that you give up coffee altogether if you like it. A cup of hot coffee after meals may help your digestion. This is a matter for your personal judgment.

If you do want coffee, I urge you not to mix it with cream. The albumin of the milk precipitated in the stomach with the chlorogenic acid of the coffee coagulates into lumps which can easily cause pains and even nausea. I have often seen on barium X-rays of digestive tubes how much more quickly the stomach disposes of milk and coffee taken separately than it does a mixture of the two. If you take milk with your cereal at breakfast, and then a cup of coffee afterward, you have nothing to fear: the milk will have coagulated with the starch of the cereal before the coffee can get in its evil work.

Cookies, see *pastry*

***Corn

P   F   C
12   9   64   calories per ear of sweet corn.

The amino acids in the proteins furnished by corn are somewhat less satisfactory for the human body than those furnished by wheat. If you eat corn bread regularly (it has approximately the same caloric values as white wheat bread), you should increase your intake of animal protein slightly, to make up for the deficiency. If you ate nothing but corn bread, you would be depriving yourself of vitamin B3 or PP and laying yourself open to pellagra. As long as you keep your diet well balanced, there is not the slightest danger of this and you can eat all the corn you want, in whatever form you prefer.

*Crabs

P	F	C	
60	18	4	calories per 3 ounces of crab meat.

See *lobster*.

**Cream

P	F	C	
4	27	4	calories per 1 tablespoon of light cream.
Tr	54	4	calories per 1 tablespoon of heavy whipping cream.
4	18	4	calories per 1 tablespoon of half and half.
Tr	18	4	calories per 1 tablespoon of sour cream.

Cream is an excellent source of fat-soluble vitamins. It usually presents no problems of digestion, but like most fatty foods it is best avoided around periods of intense effort.

*Cucumbers

P	F	C	
Tr	Tr	8	calories per 6 slices.
4	Tr	28	calories per 7½-inch cucumber.

Cucumbers are notorious for their ability to make you burp, and if they do, you had better eat them only sparingly. There is a superstition which says that they are more digestible if they are not peeled, but this is only a superstition.

*Dates

P   F C
16   9 420   calories per 1 cup, pitted.

Dates are very rich in potassium, and are fine when you need a big bundle of energy in small form.

*Duck

P   F   C
86   74   0   calories per serving of 100 grams (3½ ounces).
86   47   0   calories per serving of 100 grams wild duck.

Duck is too fat for a steady diet. Save it for special occasions.

**Eggs

P   F   C
24   54   Tr   calories per egg, raw or boiled.
28   72   4   calories per egg, scrambled with milk and fat.

Eggs have a 14% protein content, and they contain the best-balanced set of amino acids of all the foods we normally eat. These amino acids are divided about equally between the yolk and the white, but the yolk contains almost all the fat, including the cholesterol which makes it inadvisable to eat eggs every day. The white is high in sodium, the yolk in iron, potassium, vitamins A, B_1, B_{12} and D.

Eggs also contain a good deal of calcium, but unfortunately it is almost all in the shell, which is of little nutritional interest.

It is a bad idea to eat eggs raw. The proteins of the whites cannot be used by your body unless they are cooked. Also, the danger of infection is much greater in raw eggs.

Many people complain that eggs are not digestible, but except in the rare cases of genuine allergy, they are actually very easy for your body to absorb if (and it is a big if) they are fresh and properly prepared. If they repeat on you, it is probably because of the way they were cooked.

The best way to cook them is to poach or boil. If you want fried or scrambled eggs or an omelet, use the least amount of fat possible and don't let it get too hot; or use a Teflon pan and no grease at all. It is noteworthy that virtually nobody has trouble digesting eggs that have been mixed with flour or milk in custard, cakes, etc.

*Figs

P	F	C	
4	Tr	60	calories per fig.
16	9	520	calories per 1 cup of figs, pitted.

Figs are rich in potassium, iron and copper, and their enormous carbohydrate content can provide considerable energy in small volume. But their seeds can irritate your intestines, and the carbohydrate content is enormous.

***Fish

P	F	C	
83	1	0	calories per 1/4-pound serving of haddock.
80	3	0	calories per 1/4-pound serving of cod.
76	8	0	calories per 1/4-pound serving of flounder or sole.
90	9	0	calories per 1/4-pound serving of red snapper.
95	10	0	calories per 1/4-pound serving of halibut.
88	11	0	calories per 1/4-pound serving of sea bass.
87	18	0	calories per 1/4-pound serving of brook trout.
111	20	0	calories per 1/4-pound serving of shad roe.
80	30	0	calories per 1/4-pound serving of catfish.
93	35	0	calories per 1/4-pound serving of bluefish.
87	40	0	calories per 1/4-pound serving of swordfish.
88	40	0	calories per 1/4-pound serving of white perch.
111	72	0	calories per 1/4-pound serving of tuna.

P	F	C	
89	90	0	calories per ¹/₄-pound serving of sardines.
83	99	0	calories per ¹/₄-pound serving of lake trout.
87	108	0	calories per ¹/₄-pound serving of anchovies.
102	110	0	calories per ¹/₄-pound serving of salmon.
79	117	0	calories per ¹/₄-pound serving of herring.
86	126	0	calories per ¹/₄-pound serving of mackerel.
93	153	0	calories per ¹/₄-pound serving of pickled herring.
84	284	0	calories per ¹/₄-pound serving of smoked eel.

Fish contains just about the same amount of excellent protein as does an equivalent weight of meat. Like meat, it is easily digestible, and is absorbed almost in its entirety (95%) by the organism, leaving little waste matter. You can always substitute fish for meat on your diet.

The absolute equivalence of fish and meat, nutritionally speaking, is hard for some people to accept. A nice juicy steak *seems* so much more satisfying than the most delicious fish. Perhaps this is a hangover from primitive days when we ate the hearts and livers of our enemies to acquire their strength and courage. But from the standpoint of building up your body, the fish is just as good for you.

As you can see from the table, all the different kinds of fish furnish roughly similar amounts of protein, but there are tremendous differences in the amounts of fat.

For a training diet, and especially when you are approaching the Event, you should stick to the lean fish and avoid the fat ones.

***Frogs' legs

P	F	C	
48	2	0	calories per ¹/₄-pound serving.

Nice lean meat you can substitute for chicken.

*Game animals and birds

P	F	C	
96	46	0	calories per ¼-pound serving of pheasant.
95	40	0	calories per ¼-pound serving of venison.
102	63	0	calories per ¼-pound serving of quail.

Game can provide an excellent source of good lean meat if it is killed quickly and cleanly. A dying animal trying desperately to escape its doom can pump enough toxins into its flesh to make you sick.

Gelatine desserts

P	F	C	
4	0	34	calories per 1 cup.

Goose

P	F	C	
54	234	0	calories per 100-gram (3½-ounce) serving.

Goose is much too fat to be considered for anything except rare occasions.

***Grapefruit, see *citrus fruits.*

***Grapes

P	F	C	
4	9	60	calories per cup, American type, slipskin.
5	5	100	calories per cup, European type, adherent skin.
4	Tr	168	calories per cup, grape juice.

You may eat grapes at any time, but remember that they are the richest in sugar of all fruits, and therefore the most fattening. I have known women who have gone on grape orgies under the delusion that they are a diet food, and go into hysterics when they saw the results.

The skins and seeds are not very digestible, so try to get rid of them.

It is essential to eat your grapes ripe. Sour grapes will not only set your teeth on edge, they can also lead to violent intestinal convulsions. The Prussian army lost the battle of Valmy—one of the decisive battles of world history—in 1792 because of some unripe grapes. The soldiers had been marching for a long time without provisions and were dying of hunger when they bivouacked in a vineyard. They threw themselves on the grapes and suffered a mass and most inopportune onset of diarrhea. The French revolutionary army, arriving at this moment, had no difficulty in winning a glorious victory.

***Ham, see *pork*

*Heart

P	F	C
78	36	0	calories per ¼-pound serving.

Nutritive, but hard to digest. It is easy to see why heart meat is tough, it is one muscle of the body which has to work all the time.

***Honey

P	F	C
Tr	0	68	calories per tablespoon.

Like sugar, honey is rich in energy and is easily and quickly assimilated by the body. It has a slightly laxative effect. When you eat honey, remember that it comes out of your daily sugar ration, which in no circumstances is to go beyond 10% of your daily caloric intake.

***Horse meat

P	F	C
120	40	0	calories per 100 grams

Many people are revolted by the idea of eating the flesh of this noble animal (they have no scruples, however, about feeding it to their dogs), and in many places it is illegal to sell it for human consumption.† But if you don't

---

†And the U.S. Department of Agriculture does not include it in its list of edible foods, which does contain such other sentimental favorites as reindeer, opossum and whale.

mind the somewhat acrid taste and have no sentimental objections, it is an excellent lean meat which can be cooked like beef and replace it anytime on the menu.

*Ice cream

P	F	C	
8	45	40	calories per 3-ounce serving, regular (10% fat).
6	80	40	calories per 3-ounce serving, rich (16% fat).

Its high fat content suggests using it with discretion. So does its iciness, which can have a catastrophic effect on your intestines. On the other hand, if you break training and have a particularly rich main course at dinner, ice cream makes an ideal dessert as it can speed up what might otherwise be a very sluggish digestion.

***Jams and preserves

P	F	C	
Tr	Tr	64	calories per tablespoon.

***Jellies

P	F	C	
Tr	Tr	52	calories per tablespoon.

Both jams and jellies are perfectly satisfactory ways of getting your daily sugar ration. But don't forget to count them as sugars.

Kidneys

P	F	C	
75	47	Tr	calories per ¼-pound of veal kidney.

High in nucleo-proteins, which you do not want to eat regularly. Since they do not have the nutritional advantages of liver, it is best to leave them alone.

**Lamb

P	F	C	
89	57	0	calories per ¼-pound of roast leg, lean only.
90	70	0	calories per ¼-pound loin chop, lean only.

Lamb is nutritious, but generally on the fat side. Only eat chops or leg of lamb, and be sure to trim off all visible fat (there will be plenty left over in the lean).

It should not be eaten every day. Like other young animals, the lamb's body stocks nucleo-proteins to help it grow, and too much nucleo-protein in your own grownup body will increase your supply of uric acid and put toxins in your muscles that will interfere with their efficient use.

Lard

P	F	C	
0	117	0	calories per tablespoon.

Lard is almost solid animal fat. It contains no vitamins to speak of, and it is not easy to digest; two good reasons for not paying it much attention in your diet.

***Lettuce and other salad greens

P	F	C	
12	Tr	24	calories per head of Boston (butterhead) lettuce.
16	Tr	52	calories per head of crisphead (iceberg).

Can be eaten raw or cooked. The white leaves of a head of lettuce may taste better, but the green ones contain more vitamin A and C, so it is best to mix them in your salad.

**Liver

P	F	C	
60	54	12	calories per 2-ounce serving.

Liver is a remarkably rich source of proteins and of vitamins A and B complex. Since the only livers we can eat

128

come from young animals, they are also rich in nucleo-proteins (see under *lamb*) and therefore should not be eaten too regularly. Once a week is a sensible way to get the advantages of liver without its inconveniences.

*Lobster

P	F	C	
77	20	2	calories per ¼-pound of meat.

Relatively indigestible and many people are allergic to it. But it is rich in valuable trace minerals, and if it agrees with you, and you can afford it, there is no reason not to try it from time to time. Eat it only boiled, and with nothing more on it than melted butter.

***Margarine

P	F	C	
Tr	108	Tr	calories per tablespoon.
Tr	36	Tr	calories per pat.

Margarine contains fewer vitamins than butter, but also less cholesterol, and is much superior for cooking purposes.

**Mayonnaise

P	F	C	
Tr	99	Tr	calories per tablespoon.

If you don't take too much of it, this is a perfectly acceptable form of vegetable fat.

Mayonnaise, it is said, was invented by the 18th-century French general the Duke de Richelieu, who was commanding an army at the siege of Port Mahon in the Balearic Islands. One evening his cook came to him in tears: the island was so poor that there was not a morsel of butter to be found, and how could he make a sauce worthy of a general's table. There are plenty of olive trees around, replied the Duke, and some chickens; try mixing egg yolks and olive oil. The cook ran to do so, and a new sauce was born, quickly christened the mahonnaise. It has changed spelling since but remains a convenient source of energy.

***Milk

P	F	C	
36	81	48	calories per 1 cup, whole.
36	Tr	48	calories per 1 cup skimmed.
36	Tr	48	calories per 1 cup buttermilk.

Milk, in one form or another, is a necessary food for everyone from cradle to grave. It contains protein in the form of casein, which has a well-balanced collection of amino acids; and it also supplies carbohydrates and fats. It is rich in sulphur, phosphorus, potassium, sodium, chlorine, vitamins A, B2 and (either naturally or added by the milk companies) D. And with all these riches, it is relatively low in calories.

Milk is very digestible and should not ordinarily cause any stomach upsets. Yet many people avoid it on the grounds that their systems cannot stand it, and there have even been doctors (including some on the payroll of the wine industry) who have said that it is unfit for consumption by human adults. In my medical career, I have come across very few cases of genuine allergy to milk. Often my patients' complaints could be traced to the fact that they were drinking their milk too cold, a practice which can lead to painful cramps and diarrhea. If you have a genuine intolerance for milk, yogurt or cheese will do just as well. Taking your milk with a starchy dessert or breakfast cereal may help: the casein of the milk will not coagulate in big lumps in your stomach, but in little ones which will be easier to absorb.

***Molasses

P	F	C	
Tr	Tr	52	calories per tablespoon.

See *sugar*.

Mushrooms

P	F	C	
20	Tr	24	calories per cup, canned.

Mushrooms should figure in your diet only very rarely. Their cellulose content is high, and it is a particularly coarse kind of cellulose. They are rich in vitamins B_1 and B_2, but since the usual serving of mushrooms is quite small, the amount of good to be gotten in that quarter is negligible.

The woods are full of poisonous mushrooms, and hundreds of people every year suffer ghastly pains and even die of eating them. Make sure before you eat.

Rabbits can eat mushrooms that would kill you and me, and they do not feel the slightest indisposition. An old cure for mushroom poisoning was to feed the patient a concoction of seven raw rabbit stomachs and seven raw rabbit brains—not quite so odd as it sounds, since the stomach and the nerve centers of the brain are precisely the areas which the poison attacks. There are more modern and less unpleasant-sounding treatments, but modern science has still found no antidote to mushroom poisoning

Mussels

P	F	C	
65	22	15	calories per ¼-pound.

Nutritionally, mussels are much like oysters. But the danger of pollution is much higher, and the dangers of catching infectious hepatitis probably outweigh the pleasures of eating these bivalves. Mussels pass much more water through their shells than other forms of seafood, and their beards, which sift their nutrients for them, also make convenient collection-points for viruses which can later find a home in the human eater.

***Oatmeal

P	F	C	
20	18	36	calories per cup, cooked.

See *cereals*. If you like this one, you may be pleased to know that oats contain lecithin, which is also found in human cerebral cells, the little gray cells of Hercule Poirot.

*Olives

P	F	C	
Tr	18	Tr	calories per 4 medium or 2 giant, green.

To be taken with caution, because of their heavy fat content.

*Onions

P	F	C	
4	Tr	20	calories per 6 scallions.
8	Tr	40	calories per 2½-inch-diameter onion.
12	Tr	56	calories per 1 cup, cooked.

Onions are more digestible cooked than raw. They can cause gas, so should be avoided at times of intense physical effort.

**Oysters

P	F	C	
5	2	2	calories per oyster.

Oysters provide an especially good source of trace minerals (manganese, copper, iodine, zinc). They are rich in phosphorus and in vitamins A, B complex and D. They have very little fat and somewhat less protein than meat or fish. Nutritious as well as delicious, they make a highly desirable hors d'oeuvre; but they should not be eaten too often because of their high content of purines, which can increase your uric-acid count, which can cause aches in your muscles and tendons.

It is the iodine which is their chief nutritional attrac-

132

tion; there is no other food quite comparable in this respect. This is why I recommend eating a good 18 oysters every week.

Even in the non-R months? you may ask with a shudder.

There is no nutritional reason for not eating oysters all year round, as I used to do in my childhood in Brittany. Provided, of course, they are fresh out of the sea. It is true that oysters don't taste as good in summer as in winter, but this is because of the peculiar sex life of the oyster. It is male in winter and female in summer, so it has been described as being in the pleasant position of making love to itself all year long. In the summer it is producing oyster-milk for its little ones, and this is what gives the taste which some people find unpleasant.

You can always try clams as a substitute.

*Pancakes

P	F	C	
8	18	24	calories per 4-inch-diameter buckwheat cake.

Pancakes can be substituted for toast or cereal on your breakfast menu from time to time.

***Pasta

P	F	C	
20	9	128	calories per cup of spaghetti or macaroni, cooked.
40	90	112	calories per cup of spaghetti with meat balls and tomato sauce.
36	90	104	calories per cup of macaroni and cheese.
28	18	148	calories per cup of egg noodles.

Pasta provides a relatively cheap and easily digestible source of energy. Be sure to boil it in plenty of water, drain it and rinse it in cold running water before it can get soggy.

133

*Pastry

P	F	C	
12	135	204	calories per piece of apple pie (1/7 of 9-inch pie).
12	Tr	128	calories per piece of angelfood cake (1/12 of 10-inch).
12	81	160	calories per piece of devil's food cake (1/16 of 9-inch).
20	36	144	calories per piece of spongecake (1/12 of 10-inch).
8	36	128	calories per piece of gingerbread (1/9 of 8-inch).
4	27	56	calories per cupcake, no icing.
8	45	84	calories per cupcake with chocolate icing.
4	54	64	calories per doughnut.
20	135	120	calories per Danish.
8	27	84	calories per 4 Graham crackers.
4	36	52	calories per brownie.
4	9	44	calories per fig bar.
4	18	28	calories per chocolate chip.
4	18	28	calories per chocolate or vanilla sandwich.

Most diet books tell you to keep away from these foods. But if you like them, they are a perfectly legitimate source of energy, as long as you keep them within sensible limits. Make sure to keep to simple forms; avoid the gooey, sticky, creamy kinds of pastry which are overrich for your blood.

*Pâté de foie gras

P	F	C	
6	54	3	calories per tablespoon.

This is a caloric blockbuster if taken in quantities, and if you like it you are sure to take it in quantities. Save it for New Year's Eve.

***Peaches

P F C
4 Tr 40 calories per peach (about 1/4-pound).
Highly recommended.

*Peanuts

P F C
148 648 108 calories per 1 cup.
Peanuts are extremely high in fats, and they are saturated fats, which is a strike against them. Their cellulose is also quite coarse and can be irritating to the colon. They should only be taken in limited quantities.

**Peanut butter

P F C
16 72 12 calories per tablespoon.
This is much better for you than whole peanuts, because of the absence of the coarse cellulose. It is quite fattening, so use with care.

***Pears

P F C
4 9 100 calories per pear.

**Peas, dried

P F C
52 9 136 calories per cup.
See remarks under *beans, dried*.

***Peas, green

P F C
36 9 76 calories per 1 cup, cooked.
Make sure they are small and tender. Big ones are tough and hard to digest.

135

*Pickles

P	F	C	
4	Tr	4	calories per 1 dill pickle.
Tr	Tr	24	calories per 1 sweet gherkin.
Tr	Tr	20	calories per 1 tablespoon chopped relish.

***Pineapples

P	F	C	
Tr	Tr	96	calories per 1 large or 2 small slices.
4	Tr	136	calories per 1 cup pineapple juice.

*Plums

P	F	C	
Tr	Tr	28	calories per plum.

Plums have a laxative effect. Go easy on them.

**Pork

P	F	C	
60	63	0	calories per pork chop, lean only.
91	117	0	calories per roast, 1/4-pound, lean only.
44	90	0	calories per 2 ounces cold boiled ham.

Its high fat content makes it necessary to treat pork with some care. Be sure to cut off all the fat you can; this is easier if you restrict yourself to cold roast pork and ham.

***Potatoes

P	F	C	
12	Tr	84	calories per potato.
12	9	100	calories per 1 cup mashed, milk added.

The potato is primarily a storehouse of carbohydrate, hence of energy. It has small amounts of potassium and some trace minerals.

It is also quite rich in vitamin C. But vitamin C is quite fragile, and is easily lost in the process of packing and storing and moving from place to place, so try to buy your potatoes as fresh as possible. The vitamin C can also be lost in cooking, so it is better not to peel your potatoes, the skins will help keep the vitamin in.

The only cooking processes you should consider are boiling, steaming and baking. Avoid French-fries. If you want mashed potatoes, boil them in their skins, then mash them with a little milk; don't add butter or any other fat.

**Prunes

P	F	C	
1	Tr	72	calories per 4 prunes, uncooked.
8	9	312	calories per 1 cup, cooked, unsweetened (17-18 prunes).

Prunes are very rich in potassium and should figure in your diet. Their laxative properties are well known; and they are concentrated, hence high in carbohydrates, hence fattening in large quantities.

Radishes

P	F	C	
Tr	Tr	4	calories per 4 radishes.

Radishes can be hard on the stomach, and it is best to avoid them as much as possible.

***Raisins

P	F	C	
Tr	Tr	44	calories per ½-ounce package seedless raisins.

Rich in potassium, as well as concentrated energy.

*Raspberries

P	F	C	
4	9	68	calories per cup.

Quite good for you, if they don't give you a case of hives.

Rhubarb

P　F　C

4　Tr　392　calories per 1 cup, cooked, sugar added.

Its very strong laxative properties should restrict rhubarb to pharmaceutical rather than culinary use.

***Rice

P　F　C

16　Tr　200　calories per 1 cup, cooked.

The white rice we eat ordinarily is almost pure starch, a rich source of energy that is very easy to digest. If you ate nothing but rice, like so many unfortunate peasants in East Asia, you would get beri-beri, for the milling process removes all the vitamin B_1 from the rice. But you can get plenty of B_1 from the rest of your diet, so there is no reason to avoid this nutritious food.

***Salad dressings

P　F　C

Tr　100　Tr　calories per tablespoon, oil and vinegar or oil and lemon.

4　72　4　calories per tablespoon, blue cheese dressing.

Tr　54　12　calories per tablespoon, French.

Tr　72　12　calories per tablespoon, Thousand Island.

Oil and lemon is the best and makes a convenient way to get your vegetable fat ration every day. Vinegar is all right too, but I have observed that athletes often have a superstitious regard for lemons, and this is one superstition I can only approve of.

*Sauerkraut

P　F　C

8　Tr　36　calories per cup.

Sauerkraut has the nutritional properties of cabbage, with fewer disadvantages, since its preparation predigests it for you in a manner of speaking, and makes it easier to absorb.

*Sausages

P	F	C	
28	99	Tr	calories per 1 ounce salami.
28	135	4	calories per 1 frankfurter.
12	63	Tr	calories per 2 slices bologna.
8	36	Tr	calories per tablespoon devilled ham.

They are usually too fat and too spicy, hence relatively indigestible, to be taken while you are in training. A little from time to time, provided the fat content is not too high, can do no harm.

*Scallops

P	F	C	
69	2	60	calories per $1/4$-pound.

*Sherbet

P	F	C	
8	18	236	calories per 1 cup.

Same remarks as for *ice cream*, except that sherbet is obviously less fattening.

***Soups

P	F	C	
20	0	12	calories per cup of beef broth (bouillon) consommé.
20	27	56	calories per cup of minestrone.
36	27	84	calories per cup of split pea.
8	27	64	calories per cup of tomato.
20	18	40	calories per cup of vegetable with beef broth.
8	18	52	calories per cup of vegetarian.
8	27	48	calories per cup of clam chowder (Manhattan, with tomatoes).

32	54	88	calories per cup of bean with pork.
17	16	30	calories per cup of chicken noodle.
13	1	7	calories per cup of chicken consommé.
6	44	34	calories per cup of cream of celery.
24	72	32	calories per cup of oyster stew.
16	72	44	calories per cup of clam chowder (New England type, with milk).
9	14	38	calories per cup of cream of asparagus.

Homemade meat and fish soups are delicious, but they are inadvisable for your diet. When you start cooking them in cold water—which is the only way to get some taste into the soup—both meat and fish release peptones, substances which can disturb digestion by making the gall bladder release too much bile. If the peptones remained in the meat, they would be broken down during the cooking process, but they remain whole in the soup and pose problems for your insides. The problem is not so serious when you use canned soups, or make your own with bouillon cubes because here there has been some preliminary processing in the food factory which has started breaking down the peptones.

There is no problem at all in vegetable soup, which is easy to digest and can be of the greatest value to you. All the value is concentrated in the liquid; you can leave the vegetables themselves in or out of the soup as you prefer; their only function is to provide you with some bulk for your large intestine.

It is especially valuable at a time of maximum physical effort. At such moments you tend to sweat a good deal, and sweat cannot only make you uncomfortable, but also it pours quantities of vital mineral salts out through your pores. This is a necessary part of the process of removing the impurities with which your muscular effort is loading your system; but the losses have to be made up or you will suffer a severe letdown. Warm salt water can make up for the loss, but not everybody likes the taste of warm salt water. A vegetable broth with plenty of salt in it will have the same effect, and will be much easier to get down and keep down.

*Spinach

P   F   C
20 9 24   calories per one cup, cooked or canned.

Spinach is all right in limited quantities, if your intestines do not protest. It contains oxalic acid (this is what sometimes sets your teeth on edge), and too much of this can cause trouble in your muscles and tendons. I have often had to treat patients who have come down with what I call the Popeye Syndrome, the result of taking the admirable sailor's example too much to heart and gorging themselves with spinach day in and day out. Instead of bulging biceps, they often develop typhlocolitis, an inflammation of the caecum which can easily be mistaken for appendicitis and has led, on more occasions than I like to think of, to unnecessary operations.

*Squash

P   F   C
8   Tr 28   calories per 1 cup summer squash, diced.
8   9 128   calories per 1 cup winter squash, baked and mashed.

*Strawberries

P   F   C
4   9   52   calories per 1 cup, raw.

Fine if they don't make you break out.

***Sugar

P   F   C
0   0 796   calories per cup, granulated.
0   0   44   calories per tablespoon, granulated.

141

Everyone knows by now that sugar is bad for you in many ways, though it hardly deserves all the abuse that has been heaped on it in recent years.

It is fattening if you take too much of it. But its chief sin is that in the form we almost always eat it, i.e., refined, it is completely lacking in vitamins of the B group. If you eat too much sugar, you may lose your appetite for other foods containing these essential vitamins and lay yourself open to deficiency diseases.

It is, however, much too valuable and convenient a food to be given up entirely unless there is some urgent medical reason like diabetes (or obesity). It is the quickest and cheapest source of energy for muscle and brain, and can provide up to 10% of your daily calories without hurting you: say 60 to 80 grams when in training, up to 100 in periods of intense activity. Remember that this includes *all* the sugar you eat: not just what you sprinkle on your cereal or put in your coffee, but whatever is in the desserts, candy, jam, honey, or any other sweets you take in the course of the day. Never let your sugar quota go up over 10%.

Despite a popular belief to the contrary, brown sugar has exactly the same nutritional value as white, and the same total absence of vitamin B.

Sweetbreads

P	F	C	
80	20	0	calories per 1/4-pound serving.

See *kidneys*.

*Syrups

P	F	C	
Tr	Tr	56	calories per tablespoon of sorghum.
0	0	60	calories per tablespoon of corn or maple syrup.
4	9	96	calories per tablespoon of chocolate syrup.

142

Remember to count these in your sugar ration, which must never go above 10% of your day's total.

**Tapioca

P F C
4   Tr   524   calories per 1 cup, dry.
32 72   112   calories per 1 cup, cream pudding.
Can substitute for rice or other starches.

Tea

P F C
No calories to speak of.

See *coffee*, the remarks on which are applicable here, except that since there is only about a quarter as much caffeine in a cup of tea as in a cup of coffee, you can drink more of the former without disagreeable consequences.

***Tomatoes

P F C
8   Tr   36   calories per tomato (7 ounces).
Tomatoes can be eaten at will, either raw or cooked.

It is best to eat them without seeds and skins. (You can easily peel them by putting them in boiling water for about 10 seconds, and you can then squeeze out the seeds as well.) Tomato skins are eminently indigestible and often pass untouched through the stomach and the small intestine. I have often seen patients come to me in a panic with little jars containing what they thought was raw intestinal lining which had come out in their stools, but which examination revealed to be only tomato skin.

*Tongue

P F C
57 117 1   calories per ¼-pound.
Tongue has all the qualities of boiled red meat.

*Tripe

P   F   C
87   20   0   calories per 1/4-pound.

Tripe is not easy to digest, but it is rich in cartilaginous material which the cooking process changes into gelatine. Gelatine is rich in glyconol, a valuable amino acid which among other useful properties can harden your fingernails.

***Turkey

P   F   C
70   45   0   calories per 1/4-pound
Same as *chicken*.

***Turnips

P   F   C
4   Tr   32   calories per 1 cup, cooked, diced.

Like *carrots*, they should only be eaten when young and tender. The older vegetables develop a coarse cellulose which is irritating for your colon.

**Veal

P   F   C
92   81   0   calories per 3-ounces cutlet.
92   126 0   calories per 3-ounces serving of roast.

Veal has all the nutritional properties of beef. But it also, like *lamb*, contains nucleo-proteins which are there to help the calf grow and will raise your uric-acid content if you eat too much of them. So veal should not be eaten more than once or twice a week.

***Vegetable oils

P   F   C
0   126 0   calories per tablespoon.

Vegetable oils come in two classes:
1) Those with saturated fat (olive, peanut). These

should be taken in strictly limited quantities. If you have to use fat in cooking, use these in preference to butter.

2) Those with unsaturated fat (sunflower, soybean, corn). These should be used for salad dressings. They should never be used for cooking, which would make them lose all their nutritional advantages. The "critical point" at which they start to smoke is quite low; they then produce a substance called acrolein which is irritating for the digestive tube.

***Yogurt

P	F	C	
32	36	42	calories per cup, made with partly skimmed milk.
28	72	48	calories per cup, made with whole milk.

Yogurt is milk, either whole or skimmed, which has been made to ferment by the addition of microbes after pasteurization. The nutritional value is about the same as that of milk. Its calcium may be easier to absorb, and you may find it altogether easier to digest.

VI
Food During the Event

Now we can come to the day of the Event itself.

Up to now there has been no difference in the diet I have prescribed for everyone. Whatever you have been preparing for, whether it was a friendly tennis game (assuming there is any such thing) or running a marathon or running for President of the United States, your Training Ration remains the same, just as it was described in detail in Chapter IV.

When the climactic day dawns, however, circumstances change. The very importance of the Event—the immense drain on your resources it is going to represent—demands some change in your diet. And the nature of the Event creates its own exigencies: is it a short one like a slalom race in which you could not possibly eat anything even if you wanted to, or a long one like a mountain-climbing expedition in which you must eat substantially even if you aren't hungry. Will it take every scrap of your concentrated bodily strength, like weight-

146

lifting, or will it be more a matter of address and attention, like golf? Obviously, different nutritional lines will have to be taken in all these different cases.

And finally, your needs will vary in accordance with the surrounding environment—your needs under a broiling sun will be quite different from what they would be in a snowstorm.

In this chapter I will take up most of the forms of sport currently practiced and discuss them individually in terms of any special nutritional requirements they may involve on the day of the Event.

The requirements will vary considerably, but there are some general principles which apply here as well, no matter what form the Event may take.

The first and most important is one that has been named the Three-hour Law.

This law states very simply that you must never eat a heavy meal less than three hours before the start of the Event. Failure to follow this cardinal principle can lead only to trouble. Sometimes it can lead to severe and crippling disturbances and pain.

It is easy to see why. You have only so much blood in your body coursing through all its vessels to provide sustenance for all its different functions in the digestive tract, muscles, brain, glands. When you eat a sizeable meal, the digestive tract has first call; it draws blood away from the muscles and brain to help absorb the new material that has been thrust into it. Your brain, running short of nourishment, feels sluggish. Your muscles feel tired. If you start any violent physical activity at this time, you are short of blood in the very places where you need it most. An emergency call sent through your nerves will call the blood back where it is needed, but now your stomach and intestines will be short, and therefore inadequate to their task of breaking down the food you have eaten. The results may well be cramps, nausea, violent vomiting, loss of breath, and other embarrassments and disasters.

So remember this cardinal principle. Do not have a meal for at least three hours before the Event is to start. If you are all wound up, make it four hours—or even more.

But this does not mean that you should eat nothing at all during this stretch of time. Quite the contrary. Such fasting is often recommended, but I believe it is a terrible mistake. We are dealing with three or so long, tense, vital hours, hours in which you are aware of every minute passing and often in a state of considerable excitement if not acute anxiety. When you are excited or anxious, your glands are pumping extra quantities of adrenaline into your bloodstream. The adrenaline arriving in your muscles burns up sugar you have been stocking there, and a good deal of your reserves of energy can thus disappear in those endless hours. It behooves you to see that those reserves are kept at full strength.

We have just seen why you should not think of replenishing them by taking solid food. But you can and should take some liquid nourishment which will not call too much blood to your stomach but which will enable you to keep up your vital reserves of energy.

For this purpose I recommend what I call the Warm-up Ration.

This consists simply of a small quantity (one or two glassfuls) of lukewarm fruit juice, fortified with a couple of teaspoonsful of levulose or honey. You should take this every hour, or every hour and a half, before the Event; beginning about half an hour after your last meal and making sure to take the last glass no later than half an hour before the start.

What kind of fruit juice? The best in my experience has proved to be a mixture of half citrus fruit (orange, lemon, tangerine, or grapefruit) and half some other fruit like apple or grape.

Citrus fruits are quite rich in potassium and calcium, and particularly in vitamin C, which has been called the "vitamin of effort." All of these are important for maintaining your neuro-muscular balance. Your body tissues tend to acidify after muscular effort, and acidification leads to fatigue. Citrus fruits when they are burned for energy, leave an alkaline residue which counteracts the acidification, and hence are highly desirable. But taken pure, they can sometimes upset your stomach, so I find it advisable to mix them with other, sweeter fruits, which will make them pass more easily.

While the fruit juice is bringing you this assistance, the levulose or honey added to it is providing you with a supply of sugar which will quickly be deposited in the form of glycogen in your muscles, where it can be turned into energy the moment you need it. The reason for the levulose (which is the form of sugar found in honey and fruits) is that gram for gram it provides you, in comparison with other forms of sugar, with the biggest supply of glycogen. At a time when you don't want to overload your stomach, it is the most concentrated form of energy available.

A small quantity of a liquid like this Warm-up Ration should not upset your digestive system in any way. But a word of caution is in order. The only way to be sure it will not upset your system is to try it out and find out for yourself. Don't wait until the day of the Event to discover if your stomach is receptive to the Warm-up Ration. If you are a particularly anxious or nervous specimen, there is the risk that your pyloric valve might squeeze itself shut, refusing to permit the liquid to pass from your stomach into your intestines, and you would have to spew it up. It would be most unsettling to discover such tendencies on the part of your pyloric valve on the day which is of such importance to you. You should try out the Warm-up Ration well in advance, taking small quantities of it on days when you are training particularly hard. If your system takes it without protest, you can use it confidently on the big day, and it will do wonders for you in the way of sustaining your energy level.

So much for the Warm-up Ration. Now, how about the more substantial food you will need before the start of that three-hour-or-so waiting period? What kind of meals should you have before the Event, and when should you have them?

The principle is to take a copious, nourishing, well-balanced meal between three and four hours before the start of the Event. You must arrange your day's eating around this central pillar. Let us call it the *Pre-game Meal*.

It will be bigger than an ordinary meal, because this is a bigger occasion. The following is my model menu, containing what I believe to be the proper combination of two indispensable factors: easy digestibility and the provision of a good stock of energy. The meal should contain:

- 1 bowl of cereal with milk and plenty of sugar (the equivalent of 3 lumps)
- 1 or 2 toasts with honey or jam
- 1 or 2 buttered toasts
- 1 serving of freshly ground beef, heavily salted (throw in between $1/4$ and $1/2$ teaspoon), with an egg yolk beaten into it, cooked in an absolute minimum of fat. (Cooking it in a Teflon skillet or wrapping it in aluminum foil and putting it in the oven will avoid using any fat at all.)
- 1 serving of lettuce or other raw vegetable salad, with lemon juice and oil (corn or sunflower oil, preferably) dressing
- 1 or 2 ripe fruits
- A cup of sugared coffee or tea, if you are up to it. This item is strictly optional. It is best to go easy on caffeine, which is a stimulant of the nervous system, and an athlete or anyone else on the verge of a big Event is apt to be a bundle of nerves already, without need of outside assistance. If caffeine

brings on trembling, palpitations, anxiety, general agitation (all of which it is perfectly capable of doing), you will naturally avoid it.

(If you prefer, instead of the bowl of cereal, you can take a serving of rice or pasta with the meat course.)

This meal provides you with a good stock of ready energy for the trials ahead. It also gives you a fine collection of amino acids of high biologic value in a particularly digestible form.

Every item in it has its own good reason for being there. I choose chopped meat, for instance, because it has in a sense started the digestive process for you before you put it in your mouth. A hamburger will go through your stomach in half the time it would have taken in its original form as a steak.

The large amount of salt I suggest putting in the meat—it should be at least two and anywhere up to four grams (half a teaspoon)—is desirable to give you a good stock of minerals which your muscles will desperately need in the hours ahead.

You should find the meal as a whole agreeable and easy to get down. The next question is, When do you get it down?

Let us say that the Event is to start at two in the afternoon. The Three-hour Law forbids you to eat at your normal lunch hour, so the schedule of the day has to be rearranged. You should take a very light breakfast when you get up, perhaps no more than a cup of coffee or tea with two lumps of sugar. Then you will take your Pre-game Meal in time to finish it before eleven o'clock.

Suppose now the Event takes place in the morning. In this case make sure to get to sleep early the night before (with a mild sleep-inducing pill if necessary), and get up early too, at five o'clock or earlier if you have to. Suppress your usual breakfast entirely, and take the Pre-game Meal instead when you get up, taking care, of course, to leave

151

the usual three-hour interval between the end of the Meal and the start of the Event.

If the Event takes place in the evening, you will take the usual breakfast and lunch of your Training Ration, at the usual hours. Then take your Pre-game Meal at four or five in the afternoon, or whatever time gives you the necessary three-hour respite.

Another and more difficult situation arises if your Event does not take place all at once, but is spread more or less intermittently through the day.

Suppose, first, it is divided in two: you have to perform once in the morning and once again in the afternoon. This is a situation that may often arise in swimming, rowing, and track and field meets. What do you do then?

You will start as indicated previously for a morning Event. You take a Pre-game Meal when you get up, and the Warm-up Ration while you are waiting for things to start. Immediately after the morning Event is over, be sure to drink plenty of water, light mineral water if possible, a quarter to half a liter of it. Make sure that it is not too hot or too cold; the temperature of the surrounding air is best.

Then find out how much time you have till your next appearance in the cycle of the Event. If you will be able to fit in a meal more than three hours before that appearance, you have no real problem. You can have a normal meal as you would if you were following your Training Ration. If you have meat at this meal, it would be advantageous to have it chopped—you will digest it more quickly.

Take this meal about half an hour after the end of your first performance, and, of course, follow it with regular doses of the Warm-up Ration in the afternoon.

If time is limited, and you don't have three hours to digest a meal, you are faced with a dilemma, and there is no entirely satisfactory solution. You need nourishment, but you cannot afford to enter the afternoon Event with an overloaded stomach. You must have a meal, but it should be as light as possible, and mostly, if not entirely, liquid. Here is one suggestion:

Reconstitute 50 grams of powdered milk, and bring to boil.

Pour in 30 grams of tapioca, and let simmer for five minutes.

Remove from fire and add 10 grams of honey, then 30 grams of sugar.

When it is lukewarm, add 10 grams of protein powder dissolved in half a glass of water, one gram of tricalcic phosphate, one-half gram of gluconate of potassium.

This makes a drink which is a powerhouse of energy (510 calories, of which more than 92% are carbohydrates). You should take along with it

    30 to 40 grams of Swiss cheese
    50 grams of raisins, dried prunes or apricots
    3 dry biscuits

There is another category of Event, one in which you may have to appear several times in the course of a morning or afternoon, with an indeterminate wait between appearances. There is no question of taking a regular meal, but since the Event may extend over several hours and involve considerable strain and effort, you will need some kind of substantial nourishment.

A primary aim is to get some kind of easily assimilable carbohydrate into the system to meet its considerable energy requirements. The best form of carbohydrate for this purpose is glucose, since it does not taste too sweet and is less likely to create thirst. You should take 10 grams (two teaspoons) of glucose every hour or every half-hour in one-eighth or one-quarter of a liter of lukewarm fruit juice, fortified with one-half gram of gluconate of potassium, a gram of salt and a gram of tricalcic phosphate. In addition to its supply of energy in the form of quickly assimilated carbohydrates, this drink takes care of your needs in sodium, chlorine, potassium and vitamin C, and combats any tendency to overacidity in your system.

But you need more than instant energy over this long period. It is also advisable to receive some reinforcement on the protein and fat fronts. They obviously have to be in a form which can be quickly digested. I have developed a meat patty for use by bicycle riders in France—they have to eat it while in the saddle so it has to be easy on the stomach—and I suggest you take one of these patties (one every three hours if the Event stretches out interminably). Here is how to make one. Chop up:

> 40 grams of beef
> 20 grams of liver
> Mix half a teaspoon of flour with
> An egg yolk and
> A teaspoon of butter or (preferably) corn or sunflower oil

Cook for fifteen minutes in a moderate oven. Wrap in aluminum foil when cool.

To give yourself a little extra fat, you should take 20 grams or so of peanut butter or almond paste along with the patty.

This food can be absorbed quickly and easily by your body, and will give you plenty of amino acids of high biological value and also some essential fatty acids, which will be invaluable in keeping your sugar count stable and in preserving good muscle tone.

Many athletes get so tied up in knots that they claim they cannot take any food whatsoever in between successive performances. This is a very perverse attitude, because not only have their reserves been depleted in the first performance, but they are also being depleted still further by worry and anxiety while waiting. It is not too easy to talk anyone out of this frame of mind, and in some cases there is simply no use arguing. But I have found that most of those who claim they can eat nothing can actually be talked around by slow degrees. First I give them some plain water, and generally they will take this when they won't touch anything else. Then I try them on water with a little sugar in it, then water enriched with a little fruit juice. Little by little, they find to their astonishment that they can keep something down after all. And so I gradually lead them to the point where they can eat a correct ration without getting upset about it. Once they have noticed how much their performance is improved thereby, they need little more preaching on my part.

I have now laid down all the general principles you need to know for the few crucial hours immediately preceding the Event. I think the simple meals, with ordinary foods, which I suggest, will prove in the long run far preferable to any attempt to tinker with your system by cramming it with unfamiliar materials at the last moment.

Authorities and pseudo-authorities have experimented—far overexperimented in my opinion—with dietary gimmicks designed to give a momentary boost to athletes shortly before the start of their competitions. In the long run none of these gimmicks has received either serious scientific testing or universal approval, and whatever temporary good they may have been reported to do in isolated cases is far outweighed, it seems to me, by the potential dangers they represent for the organism.

In 1936, when proteins were in favor, when it was believed that meat made muscle, the American teams at the Olympic Games in Berlin were fed a superprotein diet on a scale probably unequalled since the days of the Roman gladiators. They ate, it is reported, up to 15,000 calories a day, a true Superman ration, including more than two pounds of meat. And just before they trotted out into the stadium, they were given egg yolks, sweetened concentrated milk and meat juice. Led by the great Jesse Owens, they went on to win almost every medal in sight. I shud-

155

der to think of what they might have done if they had been fed more intelligently.

Nowadays it is generally recognized that a great mass of extra protein on such a scale does absolutely no good and the task of getting rid of it puts quite a strain on an already overtaxed organism. Modern researchers, therefore, have turned in other directions. Some of them, impressed by the fact that carbohydrate is the quickest and easiest source of energy in our food, have experimented with massive doses of it. A popular system worked out by the Norwegian doctor Hermansen calls for the athlete in training to fast for one or two days, then exercise very hard while absorbing large quantities of sugar. The idea is to furnish extra stocks of glycogen in the muscles, which will be available the instant they are needed. Microscopic inspection of muscle tissue is said to have shown that increased stocks are indeed made available by this method. This may well be so. But we run into the usual difficulty on this kind of test: how well were the subjects of the experiments being fed before the experiment began? If they had been eating correctly beforehand—if they had been following my Training Diet—I am sure they would have been found to have all the glycogen they could properly take care of, stocked away in their muscles. Feeding them any more runs into the basic physiological fact that there is only a limited amount of carbohydrate the body can stock as glycogen and use directly as energy. The rest must turn into fat. So I would beware of any heavy sugar doses in a properly fed body: the last thing you want at the moment of the Event is a quantity of extra fat around your middle.

It seems to me ridiculous to shake up the eating habits of a finely tuned organism just to add what at best can be only a minute quantity of muscle tissue. It is against nature, and nature will generally find ways of fighting back. Your body may rear up and object to abrupt and arbitrary changes in its eating habits, and the possible disturbances resulting will far outweigh any marginal improvement in performance that may be reported from time to time. Coaches and trainers and athletes who have experimented with glycogen-loading are by no means unanimous in approving it; some of them say it has no effect at all.

My private opinion is that it is so much simpler just to eat well to begin with.

Another proposal which has received serious attention in recent years is to suppress solid food entirely.

In one version proposed by four American doctors, the athlete on the verge of his Event is fed intravenously with the liquid diet used in hospitals for post-operative patients. The theoretical justification for this bizarre procedure is that it takes so long for a meal to be completely digested and absorbed in the body, that half or more of the athlete's last meal may be sloshing around in his abdomen while he is running around on the field, leading to all manner of discomfort, if not cramps and nausea.

This is the kind of reasoning which appeals to all too many nutritionists. Here is a nice scientifically balanced meal of which every last drop must go directly into the bloodstream, without losing time in the long and tricky digestive process. And there is no chance for the subject's individual tastes to foul up the purity of the process. He cannot push aside a piece of meat he does not like, or sneak in an extra surreptitious bite of cherry pie. It sounds ideal.

This, like so many other ideal proposals, I think is largely nonsense—just another effort by busybody man to complicate the ways of nature, which are complicated enough to begin with and should be left alone as much as possible.

In the first place, I am not at all sure that the food injected in liquid form is really the equivalent of the meat, milk and so on going down your esophagus in the normal way. It may be a *chemical* equivalent, the chemical for-

157

mulas may be identical, but we really don't know everything about the nature of the food we eat, and it may well be that there are some qualities in meat and milk in their original state which cannot be isolated in a test tube and therefore are not present in the chemical substitute.

For another thing, the nutritional needs of athletes are not precisely the same as those of post-operative patients in hospitals. In my view, the liquid ration used for those patients does not contain enough fats or carbohydrates for someone who is going to do serious muscular work.

In addition, I believe the theoretical justification rests on a misconception. There is no reason to believe that solid food must remain an inordinate length of time in your stomach. It is a question of eating the right kind of solid food. I have taken barium X-rays of athletes after they have taken my Pre-game Meal, and in all cases the food could be seen to have been thoroughly digested between the end of the Meal and the start of the Event.

In short, I see no excuse for such violent disruption of normal processes. Not to speak of that fact that some, indeed many, people do not at all like the idea of being fed with a needle; and this is hardly calculated to improve their performance.

My disapproval is more moderate when it comes to the less radical proposal to replace the solid meal by a liquid one that can be drunk instead of being injected.

This may be indeed necessary in some cases, where eating food in the ordinary way is impractical or impossible. Recently, for example, a Frenchman named Michel Rousseau broke the world record for consecutive swimming by going back and forth in a Paris pool for 24 hours. He obviously could not take any solid food while he was doing that, and he needed nourishment. His doctor was a student of mine, and he arranged to feed him at regular intervals with a liquid constructed according to my principles for a balanced meal, except that the proportion of carbohydrate was increased to 60% to provide extra ener-

158

gy for the extraordinary muscular effort. As millions of television viewers could see, he ended up the Event (or Ordeal) in fine shape.

Events on the order of swimming nonstop for 24 hours are, however, rare. And so are the occasions where a liquid meal is required. If you really like that sort of thing, it is perfectly adequate. But under normal circumstances, why forgo the pleasure of a normal, appetizing, easily digestible meal, of the kind I have suggested? God gave us teeth for a purpose and we might as well use them.

The single Pre-game Meal I have proposed is good to prepare you for any kind of Event, and there is no need to change it significantly in any way, except in certain unusual weather conditions.

If your Event, for example, is taking place on a very hot day, or in an overheated building, you should take even more salt than indicated above, because you will be sweating it out at a much faster rate than usual. You may take up to five extra grams in the form of salt tablets.

If on the other hand the Event is to take place at a very low temperature, you will need a little supplementary fat. Simply put some more butter on your toast during the Pre-game Meal. And half an hour before the Event begins, when you take your last Warm-up Ration, take a tablespoonful of something rich in vegetable fat—peanut butter, for example—along with it.

Before turning to the particular nutritional problems of different individual sports, I would like to put in a word for an individual who is very important in most of them, but rarely gets much attention, unless he makes an unpopular decision.

This is the umpire or referee. Generally he is a good deal older than the players in the game, but his output of energy is often just as great, if not greater. He is a practicing athlete himself, and his nutritional standards should be at least as high as those of the actual players. Everything I recommend for them goes for him too.

Now we are ready to consider what happens when the Event itself begins. Here, the nature of the different activities dictates differences—sometimes radical differences—in the kind, amount and frequency of nourishment you should take.

Following is an alphabetical list of common sports. I will try to help you meet your food needs with respect to each of them. Remember that my comments, in all but a couple of cases, will apply only to food you take in the actual course of the Event. Your food earlier in the day is covered by the Pre-game Meal and Warm-up Ration already described.

ARCHERY

See *Golf*.

AUTOMOBILE RALLIES

These events, in which you try to cover a precise and difficult circuit over varied highways in a specified amount of time, are more popular in Europe than in the United States, and are not precisely a mass sport over there, being fairly expensive to participate in.

But the nutritional lessons they have to offer are valuable for the ordinary citizen every time he takes his car out for more than a routine commuting or shopping trip. A leisurely drive through the country may put no particular strain on the system. But driving the vast American distances, even over the excellent American highways, can make considerable demands. People who drive, say, from New York to Los Angeles in four or five days may be expending as much energy as they would in many athletic events, and they should take this into consideration in planning what they will eat along the way.

On such a trip, you will probably be taking more coffee or tea than usual, because of the constant strain on your nerves rising from the monotony, the cramped position, the constant hazards of slippery roads and reckless driving (on the part of others, of course, not yourself). In addition to the caffeine, I recommend that you increase your intake of protein, raising it to 20% of your daily ration. This would work out to about 150 extra calories a day, all of them in the form of high-grade animal protein, to provide your nerves with the extra amino acids they need Stop this extra protein feeding as soon as you arrive at your destination.

Many people are lured into bad nutritional practices on auto journeys by the will-o'-the-wisp of making good time. They wolf down sandwiches while driving when they would be much better off stopping periodically for comfortable meals. It is less tiring, and in the long run not being tired makes for better time as well as avoiding accidents.

On long runs it is a good idea, every time you are tempted to reach for a cigarette, to reach for a cookie or candy bar or a fruit instead. (You will suppress desserts at all your meals if you do this.) Feeding a little sugar like this to your nerve cells every hour or so can help your driving no end.

Don't forget to drink plenty of water while you are driving. Many people neglect this essential practice. Stopping every two or three hours to stretch and take a drink will not lose you any time. I should not have to add that this drink should not be alcoholic, for both physical and legal reasons.

This is a good occasion to repeat what I have said before about the necessity of getting a good breakfast before starting off. Don't gulp a cup of coffee and jump into the car in the hope of gaining a few minutes; you may get into bad trouble later. A few years ago I was visiting my brother who was chief of police in Quimper in Brittany. I arranged for him to call me every time there was a serious automobile accident in the late morning hours. I was thus able to make on-the-spot examinations and I was able to determine that a good 80% of the people responsible for the accidents had a low sugar content in their blood, indicating that they had not been adequately fed in the hours preceding.

Another thing to consider on automobile trips is the strain on your eyes. This may be considerable, especially if a good part of your traveling is done at night, when the roads are emptier but the risk of accidents is no less. It is wise to prepare for this by taking a dose of 100,000 International Units of vitamin A every day for two weeks before you set forth.

Everything I have said about the desirability of good nutrition when you drive a car goes double for when you ride a motorcycle. You don't then have the protection of the magnified crash helmet which is the automobile, and not being in good bodily and mental shape can be fatal.

BASEBALL AND OTHER TEAM SPORTS

Included in this category are basketball, football, hockey, lacrosse, polo, soccer, waterpolo, etc.

Team sports differ widely in the amount of time it takes to play a game or match, and in the amount of energy that has to be expended in them. Even within a single sport, there may be significant differences in the latter: a catcher will burn up more calories than a left fielder for example, and will need correspondingly more nourishment.

They do, however, have one thing in common, from the point of view of nutrition, and that is that they allow for periodic time-outs or rest periods when the player is not active on the field and is left more or less to his own devices.

If you are playing in a team sport, you should take advantage of any lengthy break, like the half in football or any inning when you are on the bench in baseball, to recharge your system with some of the energy it has been losing at such a prodigious rate on the field. Large quantities of water and mineral salts are seeping out of your pores in the form of sweat; the sugar content of your muscles, the prime source of your energy, is dipping; your body tissues are turning acid, leading to more or less debilitating fatigue.

To counteract all these tendencies you should take, about halfway through the Event, a small glass of lukewarm water (150-200 grams) containing:

  20 grams (about a teaspoon) of glucose (or dextrose)
  1 gram (a good pinch) of salt
  1 gram of gluconate of potassium

If the drink is too salty for your taste, you can take the salt in tablet form.

The reason for taking sugar in the form of glucose at this point, as opposed to the levulose you took in your Warm-up Ration, is that glucose provides the quickest supply of glycogen to your muscles at a time when you need it in a hurry.

It is essential to make sure that this drink is neither too hot nor, especially, too cold. Nothing is worse, in these or any other sports, than to gulp down an ice-cold drink, however tempting it may look after hard exercise or in hot weather. A sudden shower of icy beverage in the stomach is the very best way of really upsetting a digestive mechanism which is already in a state of instability on account of the onset of fatigue. Iced drinks may cause the pyloric valve to open abruptly and prematurely. This would be no calamity at a state dinner, where on the contrary an ice cream for dessert might be welcome because

163

it can help get the heavy mass of the previous courses moving less sluggishly through your system. But on the playing field, it is more apt to lead to diarrhea.

BASKETBALL

See *Baseball and other team sports.*

BICYCLING

Long-distance bicycling, which is becoming increasingly popular in the United States, has long been a national sport, almost a national mania, in France and some other European countries. I have done much work with racers on gruelling runs like the Tour de France, which takes the competitors over 4,500 kilometers of every kind of rough and smooth countryside for 20 days in mid-summer. Long association with them has enabled me to work out what I consider optimum rations for anyone who takes up biking seriously.

These rations were created for riders who are in the saddle all day, who need food that can be eaten while they are pedaling, at a time when they have difficulty getting up normal amounts of saliva (it tends to thicken during periods of intense effort) and which won't get their hands sticky either; all the while it is giving them enough energy for their very considerable efforts.

If you are just taking a leisurely ride in the country, you may prefer to take your chances at a roadside hamburger stand. This can be an unfortunate chance to take. If you are going long distances over difficult and lightly traveled roads, you will find considerable advantage in the following lightweight and nourishing provisions, which you can prepare in short order the night before.

On a day's run you should take along with you two meat patties, as follows. Chop and mix together:

40 grams of beef
20 grams of liver
An egg yolk
$^1/_2$ teaspoon of flour
1 teaspoon of butter or of corn or sunflower oil

Cook for 15 minutes in a moderate oven; then wrap in aluminum foil.

Or if you prefer you may substitute for these patties a pair of cakes made according to the following recipe. Mix well:

40 grams of flour
20 grams of protein powder
A pinch of salt.

Beat a whole egg and 50 grams of sugar, and stir into the mixture 20 grams of melted butter or margarine.

Pour in the flour and cook in a Pyrex dish, 15 minutes in a moderate oven, followed by 5 to 10 minutes of low heat. Wrap in aluminum foil when cool.

Eat one of your patties or cakes about halfway through your run, and the other about an hour and a half before arriving at your destination.

In addition to this solid food you should take along two containers. One will hold a mixture of:

Equal parts of fruit juice and
Tea, in which are diluted
30 grams of glucose or 40 grams of honey
1 gram of salt

The second will hold a liquid mixture of:

Tapioca or rice
Milk
1 gram of tricalcic phosphate
$^1/_2$ gram of gluconate of potassium

Take two or three good swallows of each of these liquids every hour or so.

You should also take along small quantities of Swiss cheese, or raisins or other dried fruits, or biscuits, to nibble at along the way. They will keep you supplied with energy the way periodic stops at gas stations would take care of your car.

BILLIARDS

See *Golf*.

BOATING AND BOAT-RACES

There are many forms of sport involving boats, to suit all tastes and purses, and about all they have in common is that they take place on water. Their nutritional demands are quite different, and I will treat them separately in three general categories.

The first can be called Regatta Racing, of which the chief characteristic is that your activity is generally limited to a single day.

The second is Deep-sea Yachting, which may keep you away and busy for days or even weeks.

The third is River-boating.

Let us start with Regatta Racing.

Regatta racing

This calls for intense muscular activity during a good part of the day, activity which may consume some 300 to

500 calories an hour. As the effort may go on for hours on end, you will have to ingest a substantially greater number of calories than you would do on an ordinary day. How do you get them?

The Pre-game Meal and Warm-up Ration described previously are sufficient to get you off and away.

But you do not want to stop there. In the excitement of a race it is easy to forget to take any liquid nourishment, but it is a serious mistake to do so. Sailing a ship is hard work and demands some extra source of energy.

What I recommend is to take—every half-hour or so, or when you can catch the opportunity—the equivalent of a glassful of a nutritious drink composed as follows (ingredients for preparing a liter):

> Equal parts of
> Fresh fruit juice
> Light mineral water
> Light tea
> 50 grams of glucose
> 1 gram of gluconate of potassium
> 1½ grams of tricalcic phosphate

There are several ways of storing this liquid. It can be kept lukewarm in a thermos bottle. It can be put in a container which is securely fastened some place where it can be easily reached, stoppered by a cork with a rubber tube going through it so that you can take a swig as you pass by. Or you can keep it in a rubber container worn under your sweater or life-jacket; in which case your body will keep it at just the right temperature, and it is always at hand when you feel the need for it.

In addition, you may have to plan for a meal on board. There may be a race in the morning, and another in the afternoon, with a variable lapse of time between. Since you have no way of knowing in advance how much time this will be—you don't know for sure how long the first race is going to take—and since you may not find it easy to get ashore between races, it is advisable on all counts to have some kind of nourishment on board with which you can replenish your depleted stocks of energy. I suggest that you keep two plastic containers on board, well lashed and easy to reach, containing the following ingredients:

In the first, a mixture of:

Equal parts of
Light tea
Fruit juice
30 grams of glucose
40 grams of honey
1 gram of salt

In the second:

Cooked rice or tapioca
Milk
1 gram of tricalcic phosphate

The two together make a nourishing meal which you can take with a minimum of inconvenience and which will provide you with a good boost of energy.

Long-distance Yachting

At first glance it might seem that the problem of getting fed on the high seas is quite simple, since there is room on board for plenty of supplies, and there is a galley to cook them in. But appearances are deceptive; as every experienced yachtsman knows, bad weather and high seas can make those supplies somewhat hard to get out, and somewhat less appetizing when you do get your hands on them.

However, it is perfectly true that in fair weather there is no problem. No matter how long you are at sea, you go on eating the Training Ration, the diet that was described in

Chapter IV. But because you are performing extensive and often exhausting physical activities, you will need more food, another 500 to 1,000 calories a day to make up for the added effort. These added calories will be divided just the way your basic ration is: 15% protein, 30% fat, 55% carbohydrate, including, if you wish, an amount of alcohol which is in no case to go beyond 4% of your total daily caloric intake.

I emphasize the latter point here, for I have often been struck by the immense quantities of liquor I have seen hoisted on board yachts which were about to go racing. This represents a great deal of money spent for what are bound to be negative results.

For too much drink will not help you sail a boat any more than it will help you hit a golf ball 300 yards or run a four-minute mile. The common misconception that alcohol warms you up is at the root of much of the trouble. I have heard yachtsmen who, judging by their way of life, seemed staunchly anti-communist, turn to the Russians for support: "Look at all the vodka they put away," they say, "to see them through their long cold winters." The difference, which seems never to have occurred to these intrepid mariners, is that the Russians do not drink all that vodka while furling sails in the icy blasts of an Atlantic gale. They drink in overheated rooms, and one reason for the overheating is that too much vodka (or brandy or any other strong drink) literally chills the blood.

Keep your booze count low, stick to a properly balanced alcohol-poor diet, and you will do fine all through the sunny days. Problems enough will arise as soon as the weather turns nasty, and you want to be in good shape to face them.

If the form the bad weather takes is cold and damp, then your top priority is to keep yourself warm, especially your extremities—head, hands, feet. The next is to add some fat to your ration. You can take 25 or 30 grams of peanut butter with each of your meals, giving you a good

169

source of the fatty acids which help the body regulate its temperature.

Your greatest need to eat is when the sea gets rough because the demands on your body are then the greatest. It is also the time when it is most difficult to get fed. The increased complexity of every maneuver on board, the constant effort of the crew on deck to keep their footing and avoid the breaking seas, the nervous tension of those trying to get some rest on their restless bunks, the heroic athletic exploits of the cook and equally athletic exploits of the would-be eaters of his fare—all these can cause a tremendous depletion of bodily energy at the precise moment when it is most difficult to do anything about it.

The general rule of the sea is to make do with what you can: a biscuit, a fruit, a crust of bread, a can of whatever you can put your hands on. You deserve more, and more balanced, food than this. If you want to, you can try the products available on the market which contain the equivalent of a balanced meal in powdered form. Look at the list of ingredients on the label to make sure they are balanced in something like the way we approve: 15-30-55. This powder tastes better when dissolved in hot water, but if you have to make do with cold you are still getting a sufficient quantity of calories in the right proportions to see you through the storm successfully.

Another great problem on the high seas is seasickness.

Since its causes are psychic as much as physical, a nutritionist can only offer a few useful hints. It is best for you to follow your own instincts when this unpleasantness starts—assuming, of course, that it leaves you enough strength and inclination to recognize and follow an instinct.

Some people claim they can control seasickness by eating heavily. More power to them. Others have a large variety of more or less magical devices for warding off the horror, and if they work for you, don't try any further experiments.

The average sufferer, however, soon loses faith in his own magical formula, and sinks into a state of extreme helplessness. He needs moral support, medicine, and a warm bed. The best that can be proposed on the nutritional front is a few sips every quarter of an hour of the mixture described earlier under Regatta Racing:

> Fruit juice
> Water
> Tea
> 50 grams of glucose
> 1 gram of gluconate of potassium
> $1\frac{1}{2}$ grams of tricalcic phosphate

That, and a little prayer, may help things out a bit.

Assuming that you are not incapacitated by this hazard of the deep, here is a model menu for a day at sea:

- *Breakfast:*
  Cereal with milk
  Tea or coffee with sugar
  Toast with butter, honey or jam
  If possible, fresh fruit and fruit juice
  If you feel the need in preparation for a strenuous day's effort, cheese, eggs or meat

- *Midday and evening meals:*
  Raw or cooked vegetable, or vegetable soup
  Cold or hot meat; or ham; or eggs
  Potatoes, pasta or rice; alternating with cooked vegetables
  Cheese or milk-based dessert
  Raw or stewed fruits

- *Midafternoon snack:*
  Tea or coffee with sugar
  Dry biscuits
  Dried fruit: raisins, figs, dates, apricots, etc.

- *While on watch:*
  Any warm drink you want, with plenty of sugar
  Gingerbread, biscuits, bread and butter

You should, in addition, take a minimum of two liters of water every day. In hot climates take two extra liters of water containing four grams of table salt and two grams of gluconate of potassium. You can take salt tablets if the taste of the salted water is disagreeable.

River-boating

Conditions are much the same as in Regatta Racing. But there is the complicating factor that you may well be in for a few, or even many, spills, usually in water that is quite cold if it is not positively icy. Once you get back in the boat, you need a rapid boost in energy to make up for what you have lost fighting the cold.

You should have, securely fastened to the boat, a plastic container filled with a mixture like this:

200 grams of tea and 100 grams of meat ground in a
    mixer. (If it is hot weather and you are afraid the
    meat may spoil, use a protein powder.)
200 grams of fresh fruit juice
50 grams of honey
50 grams of almond milk

A few mouthfuls of this mixture will do wonders in counteracting the effects of the cold.

BOWLING

See *Golf.*

BOXING

The regulations, as well as common sense, do not allow you to take any nourishment during a boxing match. It stands to reason that you do not want food in your stomach at a moment when powerful blows are being directed against it.

The regulations also call for weighing in about ten in the morning. Since boxers have to watch their weight carefully to make sure they do not leap out of their class, they do not in general eat anything in the early morning.

Since most boxing matches take place at night, it is on the whole best to hold off on breakfast till about one in the afternoon. This will hold you for a while, then, about three or four hours before the gong, you should take a regular meal, either the Pre-game Meal or a substitute like this:

A salad with oil and lemon juice
A salted chopped steak with an egg yolk beaten in
One or two pieces of toast
30 or 40 grams of Swiss cheese
Two ripe fruits

Then, every half-hour till the bout starts, a half glass of the Warm-up Ration (fruit juice and honey or levulose).

This should be sufficient to bring you in good shape to the beginning of the fight.

A subsidiary nutritional problem comes up in connection with boxing (as with other sports like wrestling, judo, weightlifting, as well as horse racing). This is the result of competitors being classified by weight. Once you are in a category, you want to stay in it, up toward the upper limit if possible, but still within it. This is not always easy to do.

There are really two separate problems here: you can weigh too much, or you can weigh too little.

Take the first case. The important thing about being overweight is not to wait till the last minute to find out about it. It makes no sense to have to go on a crash diet, spend debilitating hours in a steam bath, perhaps take pills which may be dangerous for your health in the long run, just at the moment when you should be in top form for the trial ahead. You should be devoting your full attention to it and not to the scales you will have to stand on. In addition, if you are overweight after a prolonged period of training, it means that you have been wasting time and effort carrying around unnecessary fat.

Instead of trying to do everything at the end, it is so much simpler to go on a steady well-balanced diet from the very beginning of your training period: the Training Diet I have been constantly proposing in this book.

If you are considerably overweight at the start of training, and feel you have to get down in a hurry, it is easy to lose weight by the reducing diet I have already described. It is worth repeating here:

All you want in the way of
Lean red meat, broiled or roasted or boiled,
    and served without gravy
Roasted or broiled chicken (without the skin)
Broiled or boiled lean fish (cod, haddock, sole,
    brook-trout, etc.)
Green vegetables, steamed or boiled
Salad greens, cooked or raw (with lemon juice or
    vinegar)
Skimmed milk
Limited daily portions of
A tablespoon of vegetable oil
A tablespoon of butter
1 apple
1 citrus fruit
3 to 8 lumps of sugar
1 yogurt

25 grams of cheese
Boiled eggs—3 a week
Oysters—a dozen and a half a week

Take as little salt as your appetite can bear. And drink a bottle of water between meals.

This regimen will bring your weight down rapidly, in plenty of time to go on with your training without carrying extra weight around.

If it doesn't—if you have real difficulty in keeping your weight down to the category you wish—it is time to ask yourself if you aren't in the wrong class to begin with, and shouldn't move up to a heavier one.

You may have just the opposite problem; you may be underweight and obliged to pull yourself up into your category. This is more difficult than taking off surplus pounds, because while it is comparatively simple to burn off useless fat it is another matter to put on useful muscle tissue.

Merely eating more meat or anything else will not do the trick. It may make muscular tissue available, but you will have to put the tissue in shape by exercise. Assuming that you are following a rigorous training program which is doing just that, it is all right—for a limited period at the start of your training—to increase your protein ration till it takes up 20% of your daily caloric total, without cutting down in any way on your intake of fats and carbohydrates. In other words, you should follow your regular ration but increase the protein. The extra protein should all be of animal origin.

Don't do it for too long. When you have put on the extra pounds you need, go back to your regular Training Diet, with no more than 15% protein per day.

I cannot let this subject go without mentioning the increasing, and to my way of thinking, extremely undesirable practice of artificially creating extra muscle tissue by massive doses of products called anabolistants. These certainly can have a spectacular effect, visually speaking. The muscles do swell, mostly because the anabolistants put water between the fibers. This does not really make your muscles any stronger or any more effective, but they undoubtedly look better and may bring a gasp of admiration from the audience, so they may have a strong psychological effect and actually improve the performance of the athlete who goes in for this practice.

However, the fact that the extra weight simply disappears when you stop the treatment indicates that it is not really improving your body. And there are possibilities of disastrous side effects. Witness the tragic case of the Finnish weight-lifter who had been taking anabolistants, and no one had bothered to tell him that while they expand the muscles they do not affect the tendons which attach the muscles to the bones. So his tendons were stretched to the breaking point by the swelling of the muscles, and one of them did break just as he was lifting a heavy weight over his head. It fell on the back of his neck, and he is paralyzed for life.

I wish that this ghastly example would be constantly in the minds of those who are tempted to take shortcuts with nature for the sake of temporary improvement in some athletic performance.

EQUESTRIAN EVENTS

Since you generally have to perform more than once in these events, you are really in the same position as the player in the team sports, and you should take advantage of the interim to take a drink of the kind recommended for between the halves of such games; to wit:

A glass of water containing
20 grams of glucose (dextrose)

1 gram of salt (replaced by salt tablets if it makes the drink unpalatable)

1 gram of gluconate of potassium

FENCING

Same remarks as for *Equestrian Events*.

FOOTBALL

See *Baseball and Other Team Sports*.

GOLF

Golf is typical of a certain number of sports—archery, billiards, bowling, skeet-shooting would be others—where coordination, concentration, precision are more important factors than sheer muscular strength. This is not to say that they do not represent a considerable drain of energy and do not demand substantial nourishment.

Golf can be a long and tiring game, though it will obviously never put the strain on your muscle tissue that a football game or a 20-mile ski race would. It is your nerves and your endocrine glands which are taking the greatest strain as you try to direct that little white ball the precise number of yards in exactly the right direction—not to mention the feelings of rage and humiliation when it goes the wrong distance to land in sand or water you never aimed at.

The best way to prepare, nutritionally speaking, for this strain on the nerves and endocrine glands is to give them a good supply of essential amino acids. We have seen previously that these are most easily found in good-quality animal protein. Golf above all is no game for vegetarians. Make sure you get plenty of meat, fish, eggs, milk, cheese; being careful just the same not to let your protein input for the day go above 15% of the total.

Many players in a long, tense game will take a cold Coke or a beer, or even wolf down a hot dog between holes. These may give you a temporary lift—the Coke has lots of sugar which can give you a burst of energy, the beer can induce confidence and even euphoria—but there are also good chances that they will upset your stomach and put your intestines in an uproar.

I think it is much more sensible to take along with you a mixture such as I recommended for mariners. To make a liter of this drink, mix:

Equal parts of fresh fruit juice
Water; light mineral water if you can find it
Light tea
50 grams of glucose
1 gram of gluconate of potassium
1½ grams of tricalcic phosphate.

The phosphorus in the tricalcic phosphate is especially important here, it helps ensure that your nerves can get their messages rapidly and effectively to your muscles.

You can carry this nourishing liquid with you in a thermos jug, or in a flask, which may give you a certain look of wickedness which can only impress your opponents as you take a periodic swig (every half hour or so) on green or tee.

If you are in a golf tournament which extends over several days, you are faced with the problem that is put to all participants in lengthy Events. You have to get rid of the toxins your body has accumulated during the day as a result of all your effort, the ashes left by the burning of all that energy in your muscles. At the same time you have to rebuild worn-out tissue and stock up with more energy for the next day's performance. This makes it very difficult to plan proper evening meals while the Event is in progress.

I will discuss this important question at length in the next chapter (*Food After the Event*).

GYMNASTICS

See the discussion of *Serial Events* on pages 152ff.

HIKING, BACKPACKING, ROCK- AND MOUNTAIN-CLIMBING

Nutritional problems connected with these activities vary according to the amount of time you spend at them. They can also be affected by the altitude at which they take place.

Let us start with the simplest situation: you go on a single day's excursion, starting and ending up either at home or in a hut or hostel where you can get normally prepared meals.

In this case you start with a substantial breakfast: -

An apple or banana
Sugared tea
Biscuits
Bread with butter and jam
A slice of ham

Then, when you are on your way—and particularly if you are climbing—you should stop every so often to nibble at these:

150 grams of dried fruits—prunes, figs, raisins, apricots

75 grams of almonds, peanuts or other nuts

25 grams of candy

In addition, you should drink 50 grams of Ovaltine or some similar product along the way.

When you reach the peak, or whatever the goal of your day's journey is, you should take a snack consisting of:

Salami or bologna or something similar

Ham

Bread and butter

Biscuits

When you get back to your starting point, you will want a recuperative snack to replenish some of the energy lost in the day's efforts:

Condensed milk

Tomato paste

Salted vegetable broth

Alkaline water

Later on you will take your normal evening meal, or as normal a one as conditions permit.

Now let us consider the case where your hike or climb is not limited to a single day but goes on for several.

You will have to carry provisions with you, and weight now becomes an overriding consideration, for you cannot afford to tire yourself out lugging around unnecessary bulk. This means you will be eating a good deal of concentrated instead of fresh food, and this in turn means that you will not be getting all the vitamins you should.

Therefore, you had better take along some vitamin C and B-complex tablets. But use them in moderation. You don't need more than two or three multivitamin pills per day.

While I know of no one who has been hurt by taking too much vitamin B, it is both useless and expensive to keep stuffing it into your stomach. And too much vitamin C can not only cause painful burning sensations in your stomach, it can also put toxins in your muscles which will make you feel deadly tired.

Here is a suggested daily ration for an extended tour; one that will not weigh you down with excess baggage and will also provide you with all the nutrients you need.

- For *breakfast* you will have:
  50 grams of powdered whole milk
  50 grams of concentrated bread
  60 grams of cereal
  2 cups of tea with
  20 grams of sugar

- *On the way:*
  85 grams of condensed milk
  70 grams of peanuts, almonds or other nuts
  100 grams of dried fruits

- *Midday snack:*
  40 grams of Swiss cheese
  2 cups of tea (with 20 grams of sugar)

- *Evening meal*
  20 grams of salami
  60 grams of cereal
  25 grams of margarine
  100 grams of concentrated bread
  40 grams of cocoa
  20 grams of sugar

It is better to skip the tea at your evening meal; it might keep you awake.

This adds up to an ample total of about 3,600 calories, a little rich in fats (32%) because of the considerable effort involved.

Sometimes you may be called upon to make an exceptional effort, like a life-saving mission in the mountains. It is essential to travel light. All the following can be wrapped into an 860-gram package (including 100 grams for the paraffin wrapping, which is unfortunately not eatable; perhaps a talented inventor can take care of that drawback someday).

80 grams of tuna in oil, or ham or beef
50 grams of Swiss cheese
175 grams of condensed milk
50 grams of cookies
75 grams of peanuts
50 grams of Ovaltine
40 grams of honey candy
30 grams of sugar
20 grams of powdered soup
20 grams of powdered lemon or orange
10 grams of powdered mineral salts to
   make a carbonated drink
10 grams of Nescafe or Nestea

Radical revisions in your diet are called for if you climb way up—to 10,000 feet and more. This is because of the radically decreased amount of oxygen in the air you breathe. When you reach this altitude you will need much less food than you ordinarily eat. In the rarefied atmosphere, all your body processes are slowed down and require less fuel. And you move more slowly too, expending less energy.

Thus you should reduce your daily caloric intake drastically, down to 1,600–2,000 for a person of average build.

In this ration the central place should be reserved for carbohydrates. They are easily assimilable, and they need considerably less oxygen to be processed in your body than do proteins and fats, hence they make a more economic use of the precious oxygen that gets into your lungs. You cannot upset your body's balance entirely by giving up fats and proteins, but you can cut down drastically on them. My recommendation for a day's ration at high altitudes is:

    50 grams of proteins
    50 grams of fats
    300 grams of carbohydrates

Since each gram of protein or carbohydrate produces four calories, and each gram of fat produces nine, this makes a total of about 1,850 calories.

You will need a great deal of water at high altitudes because of the dryness of the air. Sometimes it will take many liters of water to fight dehydration. You will need all the more because, to save weight, most of the food you carry comes in dehydrated form and you are deprived of the considerable water that ordinarily forms a good part of your solid food.

The water you drink will have to come from melted ice and snow, and will be almost completely lacking in mineral salts. Before you drink it, stir it vigorously to mix in some oxygen, which will make it easier to digest. And heavily dose it with salt on the way up (to acidify the blood) and with potassium on the way down (to alkalize it), thus maintaining a proper balance.

Eating nothing but concentrated food lacking in bulk for days on end may result in severe constipation. Agar-agar, whose mucilaginous texture makes it swell when mixed with liquids in the stomach, or some similar product in small doses (five to 20 grams a day) can take care of this problem.

HOCKEY

See *Baseball and Other Team Sports.*

PING-PONG

If it is a social game, see remarks under *Golf*. But competitive Ping-Pong can be very fast and tiring, in which case see *Tennis*.

RUNNING, JUMPING, JOGGING

Track and field events of short duration pose no special nutritional problems. We are long past the day when antelope or rabbit meat was fed to sprinters and goat (why not grasshopper?) to jumpers. There are more modern forms of this ancient heresy and many runners swear they get better results from all kinds of odd, unbalanced diets. But I stick to the guns I have been firing from the first chapter on: the best possible preparation for these as for any other athletic events is an accurately balanced diet with no supplements whatever.

On the day of the Event, you will follow the course already described: the Pre-game Meal and Warm-up Ration. If there are several heats and no time for a regular meal between them, every hour or so take the drink described on page 167 (fruit juice with glucose, gluconate of potassium, and tricalcic phosphate). You should also take during the waiting period a patty of beef, liver, egg yolk, flour, butter or oil (recipe on page 154). If the wait is very long, take one of these every two or three hours.

Complications arise when we get into the domain of long-distance performance.

For the ordinary or apprentice jogger, making a few

laps around the Washington Monument or some other landmark, no particular nutritional advice is necessary.

But more and more people are jogging these days for considerable distances. They are often proud of approaching that supreme test of endurance and willpower, the marathon.

It is advisable, therefore, to look into the special problems of marathoners. What is good for them is bound to be good for long-distance joggers as well.

The typical runner in a marathon race goes through a bodily crisis about halfway through the Event. His sugar count runs dramatically low, not enough carbohydrate food is getting to his muscles and his brain, and an intense feeling of fatigue is the result.

The logical thing is to give him some sugar, and this is what should be done, every five miles or so, all through the run. The trouble lies in finding a satisfactory form in which to present the sugar. Marathons are generally run in summer, and sugar is less easy to gulp down in hot weather than in cold. If it is allowed to melt in the mouth, it often creates an overpowering sensation of thirst. So it is best to take it in the form of tablets that can be swallowed whole without chewing. Or, if you can take it, try 20 grams of honey dissolved in a little water.

Much debate has arisen over the question of whether a marathoner should drink any water during the course of the race. A priori, I would say that it is a bad idea to load down your stomach, even momentarily, while running a race. However, some runners feel an absolutely overwhelming need for water, and for psychological as well as physiological reasons it would be foolish to tell them they can't have it. The only rule I would lay down would be: don't drink too much—not more than two liters over the whole course of the race, and not more than a couple of swallows at a time.

The long-distance jogger is of course under less pressure than the marathoner, but he should keep these observations in mind.

If you are running long distances in hot, humid weather with no wind, or only a following wind, you are running a real danger of heat stroke. This is a very serious condition, which you should be prepared to look out for and guard against.

In general, the heat engendered by vigorous exercise is advantageous for the organism: it stimulates the flow of your blood and all your neuro-muscular processes as well.

But heating your body past a certain level can lead to collapse, even to death.

If while running you find the heat becoming literally unbearable, you must do something to ward off heat stroke. You may at this point take a few swallows of quite cold water to bring down your body temperature before it soars into the danger zone.

This is the only circumstance in any Event under which drinking ice-cold water should even be considered. Ordinarily, it is bad for you because its sudden arrival at your pyloric valve can cause digestive inconveniences. But here it is worth running the risk of digestive inconvenience to save your life.

Under ordinary circumstances, any water you drink during the course of a run should be at air temperature.

SCUBA-DIVING AND FISHING

This is an activity which has received very little attention from the nutritional point of view, and I would not be surprised to learn that many of the unexplained accidents which occur can be laid to faulty eating habits. Digestive disturbances under water can have much more severe consequences than on land—they can even be fatal—so it is especially important to avoid them by making sure you follow a healthy, well-balanced diet when you follow this sport.

Remember that you are maneuvering in a strange environment, the sea, where your body lacks many of the defense mechanisms which serve it on land. When you are jumping or running about in the familiar air, your body has a variety of signals, known collectively as fatigue, to let you know that your reserves of energy are running dangerously low. But everything feels so comfortable in the sea (it is after all the womb out of which all life grew) that the signals don't get through. Stalking and spearing a big fish can be a very tiring occupation, but you may not be aware of it until it is too late. Commander Cousteau has vividly described the feeling of euphoria that can come over you in the depths, and the sudden and terrifying collapse that can put an end to it, when you find yourself with no strength left in a dark and hostile element.

Therefore, be sure to replenish your energy by taking some nourishment every so often when you come up for air. It has to be liquid of course, so that it can be absorbed almost immediately without setting up any digestive disturbances.

What I would recommend is a mixture I worked out once for a Channel swimmer. It is rich in fat, to combat the cold you will experience under water, and in carbohydrates, to provide quick muscle food. Every hour I gave my swimmer about 150 grams of a mixture of the following:

  150 grams of oil of almonds and grape seeds
  350 grams of honey
  125 grams of protein powder
  770 grams of fruit syrup

And every half-hour a teaspoon of tea with honey. All this lukewarm, it goes without saying.

187

This should suffice to keep you from running suddenly and dangerously out of energy.

SEDENTARY GAMES

These include such games as chess, bridge, poker, backgammon, gin rummy, etc.

It may seem odd to find these games listed in a book on athletic nutrition. But everyone who has ever taken part in a bridge or chess tournament, or an all-night poker game, knows the intense state of physical exhaustion in which the player is apt to find himself at the end.

Bridge players traditionally gulp gallons of coffee to combat the fatigue, poker players traditionally turn to whisky or beer. I cannot approve wholeheartedly of either.

Caffeine can stimulate, but overstimulation along with lack of carbohydrates can turn you into a nervous wreck. If you drink coffee, put plenty of sugar in it. Or eat some cookies and candy.

As for alcohol, though it may give you the feelings of combativeness and downright hostility which are often necessary in a poker game, it is definitely not going to improve your powers of calculation or strategy. The reason gambling houses give you free drinks is not to make you think more clearly.

What should you do then? Try what I have suggested (page 178) for the golf player who, like the card player, is putting more strain on his nerves, glands and brain than on his muscles. Put this mixture of fruit juice, water, light tea, glucose, gluconate of potassium, and tricalcic phosphate in a container, and pour yourself a nourishing glass every so often in the course of the long, tense hours.

SKATING

See the discussion of *Serial Events* on pages 152ff.

SKIING

The essential element affecting your nutrition when you go skiing is the length of time you spend on the snow.

If your Event for the day is one glorious downhill run or giant slalom, there is no special problem. You follow the general principles laid down at the start of this chapter, take your Pre-game Meal and Warm-up Ration, and that is all.

If you are racing more than once, or if you are going up and down the slopes all day, your problem is that of serial performances, which I have discussed at length on pages 152 to 155. You can take the fruit-juice-and-glucose drink, and the meat patties, which are described there, at appropriate intervals.

When we come to Nordic or cross-country skiing events, long-distance races, etc., the picture changes entirely.

Here we are dealing with a combination of environmental conditions (cold and altitude) and intense muscular activity which sets up enormous caloric demands, going up in some cases to 7,000 calories burned up in a single race. Some skiers refuse to take any nourishment at all in the course of these races, because of the loss of time involved. But it seems to me that, at least in races of 15 kilometers and more, a few seconds lost in replenishing your forces are little enough to give up in return for avoiding the crushing fatigue, both physical and mental, which you risk otherwise.

A Pre-game Meal should be taken, as usual, at least three hours before the race. Since the temperature is going to be cold, you should take a supplementary fat ration in the form of a tablespoon of almond paste or peanut butter with the meal.

Then comes the usual Warm-up ration of fruit juice and honey till the start.

The general practice in the past, where skiers did stop to take some food, has been to give them some carbohydrates every eight or ten kilometers in the form of warm sugared lemonade, or honey mixed with warm water or blueberry syrup; stopping at four kilometers before the end of the race.

There is no doubt that all this energy-rich sugar is valuable. But I think the carbohydrates should be supplemented by some fats and proteins as well.

My recommendation for a 50-kilometer race, for example, would be to take 100 grams of one of these sweet syrups at the 10th, 20th, 30th, 38th and 46th kilometers. In addition, at the 10th and 30th I would add a patty consisting of 40 grams of cooked, freshly chopped steak and 30 grams of peanut butter.

You will need plenty of salt too, because the air at high altitudes is dehydrated, and the extra salt will keep your body from losing too much water. Spread two to three grams of table salt and one of gluconate of potassium through these different preparations.

In fact, you ought to be stocking up on salt by taking extra quantities of it for several days before the race, along with an increased ration of water.

Finally, you may well need extra doses of vitamin A to help protect you from sun blindness. You could eat large quantities of butter and carrots and cod-liver oil; but it is perhaps simpler to take a capsule of 50,000 International Units of vitamin A every day you race.

SPELUNKING

This activity, which has only recently begun to interest a sizeable public, demands a considerable muscular effort in climbing, crawling, sometimes plunging into ice water, under most difficult environmental conditions of cold, darkness and damp. Rations have to be packed in waterproof and shock-resistant wrappings and, of course, have to be kept as light in weight as possible.

I have drawn up two rations which I think meet the special demands of this arduous sport. The first is for breakfast and for the midday meal:

125 grams of condensed milk
120 grams of biscuits
50 grams of dried fruits
50 grams of peanuts or almonds
50 grams of chocolate
20 grams of sugar
50 grams of candy
5 grams of Nestea or Nescafe

This is a ration very rich in carbohydrates (a good 64% of the total) to stoke up the energy you need for the intense muscular effort and mental strain.

This is balanced by the ration for the evening meal:

50 grams of pemmican
70 grams of ham
70 grams of Swiss cheese
60 grams of precooked pasta or rice
60 grams of biscuits
45 grams of powdered soup
20 grams of sugar
20 grams of butter
5 grams of Nestea or Nescafe

In addition, you should take small supplements of vitamin B complex, and 350 mg. of vitamin C.

If the expedition lasts several days you will have no access to liver, green vegetables or whole milk, so you will be running short of vitamin A, of which you have particular need in the more or less permanent darkness in which you are moving.

When Michel Sifre, who holds the world's record for length of time spent in underground caves, made his first spectacular performance—he was down for more than 100 days—his vision was badly impaired when he came back above ground, and for two weeks it was feared that he would be permanently blind. It was assumed at the time that prolonged darkness had caused something in his eyes to atrophy, but I suspected a dietary cause. I discovered that Sifre, who couldn't stand the taste of butter, had simply erased it from his daily ration. The next time he went down I suggested he take substantial doses (50,000 to 100,000 International Units) of vitamin A every day. He had no further trouble with his eyes.

TENNIS

Tennis can be a very vigorous game. It can also be a very uncertain one. You are lucky if you know when your match will start, and you have no way of knowing how long it is going to take. If you are evenly matched with your opponent, it can go on for hours.

If it is a long, hard-fought game, you will do better for taking some kind of nourishment before it is over. Too many tennis players content themselves with taking a between-the-sets swallow of an ice-cold carbonated beverage. Nothing is worse, in my opinion; both the ice-coldness and the carbonation are capable of disrupting the work of your digestive organs and producing inconveniences or worse: burping, feelings of nausea, even vomiting.

I recommend instead the drink I have described in the section on Team Sports (page 163):

> 150-200 grams of water (not too cold, not too hot)
> 20 grams of glucose
> 1 gram of salt
> 1 gram of gluconate of potassium

Again, if this drink is too salty for your taste, you can take the salt in the form of tablets you can swallow whole.

If it is a long hard match, you might also consider taking one-half or even a whole meat patty (its composition—beef, liver, egg yolk, flour, butter or oil—is described on page 154) in the longish interval between the third and fourth sets. This may seem like a positively horrifying notion, but it makes good nutritional sense. It is easy to digest, and it can give you some of the energy you desperately need for the last hectic moments of the match. If you eat this patty, don't forget to take the drink described above at the same time.

WATERSKIING

There are so many variables in this sport—the temperature, the humidity, the wind, the spray, the dangers of sunstroke or a douse in unpleasantly chilly water, even the relative stickiness of your bathing suit—that it is impossible to lay down any hard and fast rule as to how many calories you will need during any particular day. But in general it can be said that waterskiing counts as hard work, and you will need all the nourishment our Pre-game Meal and Warm-up Ration can give you. If you are racing twice in the course of a single day and there is not time for a regular lunch three hours before the second one, you may take the rations described on pages 167 and 168: a drink made of 10 grams glucose dissolved in fruit juice, plus a meat patty.

Or you can replace the meat patty with the following liquid tapioca preparation:

Reconstitute 50 grams of powdered milk (it is easier to get your hands on this than on fresh whole milk in a yacht basin) and bring to a boil
Pour in slowly 30 grams of tapioca
Let simmer 5 minutes without stirring
Remove from fire and add
10 grams of honey and
30 grams of sugar
When the mixture is lukewarm, add
10 grams of protein powder dissolved in half a glass of water
1 gram of tricalcic phosphate
1/2 gram of gluconate of potassium

If the weather is cold and damp, you are going to lose precious body heat through your bare skin. You should increase your consumption of vegetable fats to help counteract this. Take about 30 grams of peanut butter with your meals.

If on the other hand the weather is very hot, you will need to make up for the loss of water and mineral salts you will sweat out. You should add to one of the drinks of your Waiting Ration a gram of gluconate of potassium, one gram of tricalcic phosphate and one gram of table salt.

WEIGHT-LIFTING

See the discussion of *Serial Events* on pages 152–155.

Weight-lifters with their prodigious muscle masses may need a little more B_{12} than the rest of us, and therefore more than they get in a normal diet. A supplement of 150-200 micromilligrams daily should suffice.

VII
Food for After the Event

We have seen in the course of previous chapters what is the best diet to prepare you for the Event which is to tax your reserves and your physical and mental resources. And we have also seen what if possible you should take in the course of the Event itself, during whatever breathing space or rest period is provided by the nature of the activity.

This does not exhaust the subject, however. There is another period of primary importance from the nutritional point of view, but one that has been almost entirely neglected in the past. This is the period *after* the Event is over. What do you do when the last whistle has been blown, when the last drop of energy has been drained out, when the cheering or the groans have erupted in the stands, and it is time for the performer who has been putting his whole life on the line for all those agonizing minutes and hours to start relaxing? How do you start to

196

make up for all the immense strain to which you have been subjecting your body?

The answer is all the more important because of the immensity of the strain. Your muscles and nerves have been called on to make really extraordinary efforts, much beyond the scope and scale of your daily activities. No matter how many times you have been called upon to make it in the past, such a strain wrenches you, it throws off your bodily balances. You owe it to yourself to give them the best possible chance to get back into healthy equilibrium.

Your body is quite vulnerable at this moment of letdown. Off balance already, it can go off the rails entirely; it is wide open to infection. It is in bad need of what I call a Recuperative Ration, to enable it to resume its normal functions with a minimum of trouble.

Unfortunately, an immemorial tradition is at your elbow at this inauspicious moment to offer you some particularly inappropriate nutritional advice. Ask yourself the question, and you will probably say that once the game is over, the struggle is done, your first instinct is to celebrate the victory, or to lament the defeat, in a feast that can become a perfect orgy of food and drink.

This is a social instinct, not a physical one. You do it because everyone has always done it, or so you have been told. When the World Series is over, the television cameras follow the winning team into the clubhouse where they are breaking out magnums of champagne. It has always been like that. The most ancient literature of the most ancient peoples is full of gargantuan feasts which followed a successful hunt, a successful battle, a successful chariot race. The victor has always enjoyed the chance to show off his generosity by standing endless rounds for all his friends and supporters. The vanquished can at least hope to get his mind off the bad news by mingling with the crowd and trying to enjoy himself.

This is easily understandable, but it is not necessarily wise. When you sit down and bellow for a roast bear and a stagshorn full of ale (this is what the Vikings used to do, but it is not unlike what I have seen in 20th-century restaurants) you are letting social pressures do your thinking and bellowing for you. If you stop to check up on your real feelings, you will generally find that when you come out of an intense physical effort, you are not terribly hungry. Often quite the contrary, you have no appetite at all. Your primary physical sensation is that you are tired. Fatigue is your body's way of letting you know that your blood is full of toxic matter, the residue or "ashes" of all the energy you have burned, far more than the normal excretions of the system can get rid of in a short space of time. In the hyperactivity of muscle and gland that has accompanied the physical and emotional stress, parts of your body have been literally worn out. What you need now is to get rid of the poisonous ashes and to rebuild the body cells which you have sacrificed to your effort.

Let us see how to go about this rationally, even if it means forgoing the pleasure of that magnum of champagne.

The first thing your body needs after strenuous effort is water and salt, to replace what you have passed out in great quantities in the form of sweat. Therefore, as soon as the effort is over, you should take a glass (300 grams) of water or soda water, lukewarm or warm, containing a gram of sodium chloride (table salt) and $3/4$ of a gram of gluconate of potassium.

The reason is that the bulk of the toxins left in your body is going to be eliminated in your urine, and you want to speed up diuresis, the urine-making process. There is no doubt about the need for water—tests have shown that a drink of water after physical exercise has a marked diuretic effect as compared to simple rest. About salt, you will hear contradictory opinions. Some experts do not approve of giving it immediately after the physical

198

effort. They say you will need it sooner or later, but the sodium in the salt retains water in the body and thus delays diuresis; hence they recommend not taking salt till later. My own feeling is that after the profuse losses you have suffered in sweat, a small dose is indicated to recover your full bodily equilibrium and cannot have any deleterious effect.

As for potassium, no one doubts that you must make up for your losses immediately, for you cannot excrete your body liquids correctly without an adequate supply of potassium in the blood. If you are short of potassium, your excretions will proceed more slowly and you run the risk of spreading poison throughout your body.

Next step: after your shower and rubdown, take a glass of skimmed milk, or whole milk if your system is up to it. This provides you with some more liquid in a somewhat more agreeable form than salted water, and it also starts re-equipping you with the calcium and mineral salts you need to replace the worn-out proteins in your tissues.

Then, half an hour or so before your evening meal, take two or three glasses of water, preferably a light mineral water—your body still has a great need for liquids.

As for the evening meal itself, it should not be the feast you may have dreamed of. Maybe you can't avoid the chorus of invitations and encouragements from your dear friends, but ideally you should be taking no more than a dinner like this:

A bowl of salted vegetable broth

A dish of rice, or pasta, or boiled potatoes liberally salted and served with butter and grated cheese

A green salad with lemon juice and oil, and a hard-boiled egg

1 or 2 slices of toast

1 or 2 ripe fruits and a few dried fruits (prunes, dates, figs)

A glass of light red wine at the end of the meal (if you

really want a drink; it may not be quite in the league of the magnum of champagne but will be much better for you in both the short and the long run).

This may seem like a remarkably skimpy ration after the enormous outburst of energy you have expended. However, my experience has shown that it is ample for the average athlete. It gives you just enough carbohydrates, in the starchy food (rice or pasta or potatoes), to start replenishing your stocks of energy. (This is preferable to the common practice of taking sugar directly after the end of the effort. I find no justification for it. Although the sugar count of your blood is quite low at this point, it will re-establish itself in due time without forcing, so it is not worth fretting about.)

It gives you a smidgeon of fat (the butter and oil) but not too much—fat is to be avoided at a time like this: any fat you melted off in the course of the Event is a welcome loss, and too much fat in your digestive tract at this precarious moment may throw your whole system haywire.

You don't want to fill up on animal proteins either; they will only accumulate uric acid and ammonia in your blood at a time when you have too much of them already. That is why I recommend laying off meat entirely until the evening of the following day. The egg, cheese and milk will provide you with the minimum of protein you really need at this point.

The fruits, salad and fruit juice are there to replenish your stock of vitamin C which is vital for restoring your depleted adrenal glands and for combating the acidifying tendency resulting from fatigue.

The green vegetables give you whatever vitamin B you may need.

The hard-boiled egg and the butter provide the cholesterol you need at this time for your adrenal glands.

200

In addition, you need a recharge of vitamins B_6 *and* B_{12}, and while some of this is provided by the bread and milk, you may want to take a multi-vitamin pill as well at this dinner following the Event.

I repeat, this modest meal should be quite sufficient; it is all that your tired and bruised body really wants. At least such has been the case in the vast majority of cases I have observed during my career. It is possible that this doesn't apply to you, that you came out of your Event feeling ravenously hungry. It may be, in that case, that you weren't putting as much of yourself as you thought into the effort, and that you were therefore not really suffering from fatigue in the full biological sense of the word. Or it may be that, simply, you are an exceptional person, with a make-up quite different from the rest of us. In either case, there is no reason why you shouldn't eat all you want. Let your appetite be your guide.

But let us suppose that you are like the majority, that you are not really hungry. Then you will definitely be better off with my brief, meatless dinner.

Before you go to bed, be sure to take another glass or so of milk, skimmed or whole, to keep up your minimum protein requirements and also to make sure you are getting plenty of liquids into your system.

Still assuming that you are an average, healthy mortal and not an exception to the rule, my opinion is that your diminished appetite will continue into the following day, for it takes a good 24 hours for the body to get back into some kind of balance following severe and prolonged effort.

On this following day, you should eat a good deal less than you have been doing on your daily Training Ration. In fact, you should cut a good 1,000 calories out of your day's diet.

Here is my model for what you should eat on the day *following* the Event:

- *Breakfast:*
  A cup of light tea or coffee with 2 or 3 lumps of sugar
  2 pieces of toast with jam or honey

- *In the course of the morning:*
  A tall glass of fresh fruit juice

- *Midday meal:*
  A raw vegetable salad, with salt, oil and lemon juice
  A dish of rice, pasta or potatoes, served with butter and grated cheese
  Raw lettuce, with oil and lemon juice
  1 or 2 slices of toast
  1 or 2 ripe fruits and a few dried fruits
  A glass of light red wine if you want it

- *Afternoon tea:*
  A big cup of tea with plenty of sugar; or a tall glass of fruit juice or mineral water

Thus far, as you can see, we are chiefly interested in replenishing you with energy-rich carbohydrates and vitamins. By evening you are ready to go back to something more normal; your body can take a meal quite like that of your regular Training Ration.

- *Evening meal:*
  A bowl of vegetable broth
  1 serving of white meat (veal or chicken; easier to get down than red meat, largely for psychological reasons—they are nutritionally identical); or 2 slices of lean ham; or 2 boiled eggs; or fish
  1 dish of steamed vegetables with butter
  Some cheese
  Some ripe fruit, or stewed fruit, or a piece of light pastry
  A few dried fruits (rich in potassium)
  A glass of red wine—optional as usual

It is on the next day, the second following the Event, that you can afford to let yourself go and eat heavily. By now your body has made the necessary adjustments, and your appetite is at liberty to come back in a flood. I have repeatedly noticed this phenomenon in athletes, and my empirical observation is confirmed by a study made by four English researchers of cadets in a military academy, published in the *British Journal of Nutrition*. They made a detailed study, day after day, of the calories spent in energy and the calories taken in by food. They found a strikingly close correlation between the quantity of calories burned up as energy on any particular day and the quantity of food eaten two days later. Every time there was a rise in effort, there was a parallel rise in appetite 48 hours later.

I therefore recommend increasing your food intake drastically on the second day following the Event. You may increase your day's ration by 1,000 or even 1,500 calories. After all, your body deserves some reward for all the work it has done for you.

Here is a model day's ration.

- *Breakfast:*
    A bowl of cereal, amply sugared
    A boiled egg
    Ham; or cold chicken; or cold roast veal
    3 pieces of toast
    Butter, honey, jam
    Tea or coffee, well sugared

About 10 in the morning, take two to four glasses of water, light mineral water if available.

- *Midday meal:*
    A raw vegetable (lettuce, carrots, tomatoes) with oil
      and lemon juice

203

A portion of red meat, grilled or roasted
dish of potatoes, rice or pasta, with butter
Cheese
A rice pudding, with milk
2 fruits
A glass of light red wine

- *Afternoon snack:*
  1 glass of milk
  2 pieces of toast
  A little Swiss cheese
  1 fruit

- *Dinner:*
  Vegetable soup
  1 order of white meat—veal or chicken—or fish
  Potatoes or rice or pasta
  Cheese
  Stewed fruit
  2 ripe fruits
  A glass of (optional) light red wine

At bedtime, take a glass of light mineral water.

Then, next day, you are ready to go back to the basic Training Diet we have described in Chapter III.

All the discussion up to now has been on the basis that your Event is over and done with in a single day, and you have the following days to rest up. You can take advantage of this period: you can afford to cut down on your food intake temporarily to give your body a chance to work out its own adjustments.

This is not possible when the Event goes on for several days, as it is all too likely to do in most competitive sports these days. This calls for a completely different nutritional strategy. You cannot afford, after the first day's activities, to follow the Recuperative Ration I have been describing: it would indeed clean a good part of the poisons of fatigue out of your organism, but it would leave you undernourished and too weak for the intensive efforts of the following day or days. It is unthinkable to starve yourself on the verge of a maximum effort.

In practical life, of course, you will make allowance for this. If your Event is, say, a marathon race or a football game, you know you will be expected to give your all during the time it lasts, and you will be on your own afterwards. If it is, say, a four-day golf match, you obviously will not strain yourself to the utmost on the first day; you have to leave something over for the following ones. You will have a good accumulation of the toxins of fatigue at the end of the first day, but not to a crippling extent. And your first priority will not be to get rid of them, but to build up your reserves of energy for the next day's efforts. Any disintoxication you can perform in the process is all to the good, but for the moment this is a secondary consideration.

So you will face a situation after the first day's round of whatever it is, of being tired but not completely exhausted. You may be tired enough anyway so that you are not hungry. But unlike the circumstance when your Event is over and done with, you must this time force yourself to eat a substantial meal, to make sure that your body does not run dangerously short of its supplies of energy.

Immediately after the Event, you will want to drink about 300 grams of water, along with 30 grams of honey, one gram of salt, one-half gram of gluconate of potassium. This is exactly what you would take after a one-day Event, except for the addition of the honey, which provides a painless way of starting to replenish your sugar (i.e., energy) supply as soon as possible.

After the shower or rubdown, take (as in the one-day case) a tall glass of whole or skimmed milk.

Then, when the time comes for the evening meal, no matter how feeble your appetite may be, you should take something like this:

A vegetable soup with vermicelli

A salad with lemon juice and oil, and a hard-boiled egg (soybean shoots would make a particularly good addition to your salad if you can find them)

A piece (150-200 grams) of grilled or roasted red meat. If your Event goes on for several days, replace the red meat with 150 grams of liver every third evening

Pasta or rice and butter

Cheese

100-150 grams (4-6 slices) of bread

1 piece of pastry, preferably a fruit tart

Dried apricots, dates, prunes or figs

2 fresh fruits

A couple of glasses of light red wine with the cheese or after dinner if you like it

At bedtime, take 150 grams of fruit juice with 20 grams of levulose, which as we have seen is a good way of giving you sugar to put away for future consumption.

Such a regimen tries to serve both our principal purposes. It furnishes you with a good quantity of liquids and mineral salts to help your body make up for its losses through sweat, and clean itself of the toxins that have piled up in it. It keeps you well supplied with vitamins B_1 and B_6 (the liver), with calcium (milk and cheese), with vitamin C (fruit), with vitamin B_{12} (liver and eggs). Above all, it gives you the reserves of energy you need for the daily grind.

When the next day dawns, you will prepare for the second stage of the Event (and eventually the third, fourth and so on) exactly as you would for a one-day Event: breakfast and lunch if there is time for them, Pre-game Meal, Warm-up Ration. Then after your performance, the liquids and the copious evening meal just described.

Only after the last day's activities are over, and the Event definitely completed, will you forgo that big dinner and turn to the Recuperative Ration—the skimpy meal through the first 24 hours, the heavy ones on the second day following the end of the Event—which will return your body to its normal balance and let you resume your normal diet after three days.

These post-Event 48 hours are really the only time when you should consider a change in your ordinary well-balanced menus, and a short enough time it is, considering the violent stress and sometimes radical wrenches to which you have subjected your frame. But if you have been following the Training Ration conscientiously while you were preparing for the Event, your body should be in good enough shape to get back to normal in this brief period of time.

VIII
A Word About Sex

This is a book about the feeding of athletes, with the idea of improving their performance, or at least maintaining it on a high level.

The question may have occurred to you: does this also apply to the category which Dr. Kinsey named sexual athletes, whose feats form a continuous subject of underground anecdote and admiration? Sometimes these anecdotes get into the history books, as when we come across a figure like Augustus the Strong, Elector of Saxony, who sired 365 sons and daughters. Reputations like this are generally passed around privately, but passed around they are, and often they stir up feelings of envy. Many a man has asked himself if he could not emulate the feats of Augustus the Strong, as many a woman has asked if she could not emulate the equally fabulous ones of Catherine the Great, empress of all the Russias. Often these questions have taken a form which it seems apposite to take up in this book: will variations in diet increase the range and improve the style of sexual performance?

It is widely believed that they will, and the tradition of turning to what Lord Byron called "the amorous foods—oysters, eggs and such" seems to be as old as the human race. Antiquity went wild for brews made of the testicles of bulls. The Middle Ages saw a great vogue for the mandrake, a root with a marked resemblance to the male reproductive organ, especially when it grew under gibbets, where it was supposed to have been planted by the ejaculation that accompanies the last dance of the hanged man. The spice trade which plays such a large role in the history of navigation was partly based on the belief that spices could be used for aphrodisiac purposes. To this day in Oriental cities like Hong Kong there is a brisk trade in adders' gall and similarly unpleasant products. And it has been claimed that the African rhinoceros is in danger of extinction because of the widespread belief that its horn, when ground to powder, is an infallible prescription for potency.

In Western countries, some people simply eat more meat.

Is there any justification for all these beliefs?

I am afraid that there is not much that nutritional science can add to the discussion. Certainly sex involves muscular, energy-devouring activity; it is a physical act of greater or lesser caloric output depending on circumstances and the temperament of the people involved. If it were only a physical act, the answer would be easy. We could say that it was no different from any other form of exercise, part of the daily energetic process of the body. Lenin said something like this when he compared sex to drinking a glass of water: something you did periodically for the good of your body without thinking too much about it—a chance remark which had a disastrous effect on the emotional life of many devoted Communist Party members in the old days. In that case, we could say that sex could be put in the category of one of the different sports we treated in Chapter VI, and we could plan a nutritional approach to it accordingly.

But despite what Lenin said, sex is immeasurably more complicated than drinking a glass of water. It involves the mobilization and release of many and complex forms of energy, far transcending the simple muscular exertion involved. Muscles, nerves, glands, brain—everything is involved.

Finding the right food to prepare for this whirring bundle of energies and desires is not quite the same as finding the right meal to precede a game of tennis. Perhaps rhinoceros powder will serve you better than anything in my Training Ration.

As a normal physical activity, there would appear to be no particular reason why sex should be performed less at one time than at another. Athletes don't think so, however, and they are undoubtedly right. I have seen them again and again come by the thousands from the ends of the earth to the Olympic Games, and most of them are as chaste as nuns for days or weeks before the start of their Event.

This may be because they are paying their tribute to the ancient, probably prehistoric, superstition that in ejecting his seed man somehow diminishes his strength, while holding it in will retain his power and enable him to triumph over his foes. Physiologically speaking, this is pure nonsense, but it makes good psychological sense. A man or woman straining every effort, concentrating everything in body and mind on a single end, a single performance, cannot afford any distraction. And sex can be a major distraction; it can all too easily set up an inner turmoil that would be ruinous to successful achievement.

Once the Event is over, of course, things change dramatically. It is fascinating to watch the Olympic village change, in a few days or hours, from a monastery to a bordello. The picture is complicated by the fact that participants in some of the earlier events like rowing are ready for the change while others, like the runners and jumpers, are still keyed up to a state of purity. But one way or another, after the Event is over, the bars are down, and from one end to the other of the community, without regard to age or sex or social system, there is a tremendous urge to seek release in what used to be called the joys of the flesh.

The famous athletes I have known have all led quite active sex lives. There is no special reason to believe that they are more spectacular performers in bed than anyone else. They have less trouble than the rest of us, it is true, in picking up attractive bedmates, but that is because they are famous athletes, not because of any particular prowess in amatory techniques.

There are too many parameters to the sex act to believe that merely toning up your system with the right foods can solve all your problems.

But conversely, there is no reason to disregard the physical factor altogether. Other things being equal, you will clearly be better off if you are in good physical shape. You will be in better physical shape if you have been following an intelligent, well-balanced diet adjusted to the needs of your personal organism, in short, if you have read this book and are following its counsels.

This does not mean that you have to take it to Aspen with you for that glorious weekend on the slopes. or bring it along on your honeymoon for a periodic peek. There is a time for everything, and there is a time for ordering a fancy, unbalanced meal and a bottle of champagne.

You can always go back to the Training Ration again when you come back to the humdrum nine-to-five world of reality.

IX
Diet and Disease

Athletes are, more or less by definition, in better physical shape than ordinary mortals. This does not mean that they are less subject to disease. In my professional experience, I have often been struck by the wide variety of disorders that Olympic and professional athletes may be subject to. I am struck too by the number of these that can be ascribed, very simply, to faulty habits of eating.

I do not mean to make nutrition the center of life. Obviously, there are other factors. If you are poisoned by chemical fumes from the local refinery, if you are knocked down and break your leg, if an anopheles mosquito puts the parasites of malaria in your blood, these are events quite independent of what you may have had for dinner last night.

There is an infinity of pathological states into which you can enter and which should be taken up only with your doctor. Fortunately they are rare in the life of the normal healthy man or woman. All I propose to do here is to outline a few conditions I have often encountered, and propose simple dietary means for dealing with them. I am naturally not proposing do-it-yourself remedies for what may be serious internal maladjustments. But if you are feeling bad, it is almost always a good principle to see if you are not committing some nutritional sin and try to correct it. You can always go to see the doctor afterwards if it doesn't work.

Many digestive troubles are due simply to boredom. If you eat in messhalls or canteens, the food is apt to be depressingly monotonous. You find your appetite dulled by constant repetition of the same unattractive dishes. A natural reaction is to eat less and less of the main course. In the natural order of things, this would make you lose weight, which would be a sign that something was wrong. But the effect may be concealed because to make up for the unappetizing meat, you stuff yourself with bread, apple pie, chocolate sundaes and whatnot. Your weight may stay the same, but your diet has become unbalanced, it is running short of vitamins B and C, and the result may well be severe stomach cramps. If you suspect that this is the cause of your trouble, try to get some variety in your food; at all events be sure to balance your meals better, take a few multivitamin pills if necessary, and the cramps will rapidly disappear.

STOMACHACHES

Most stomach trouble is caused by two elementary dietary errors which I have mentioned before, and which I cannot mention too often. They have charming scientific names: *tachyphagy* and *pinotrogondia,* which mean simply eating too fast and drinking too much during meals.

Regarding the first point, I always tell my patients: remember that Nature put teeth in your mouth, not in your stomach. The point of having teeth—outside of flashing a

Fawcett-Majors smile—is to chew your food. If you don't chew it enough, you are putting an extra unneeded burden on your stomach, asking it to perform work that should have been done by your salivary glands. Faced by such a burden, your stomach does its best by increasing its secretions. This means putting more acid in your stomach, and acid burns. You know the feeling. And even so, there may not be enough secretion to handle all the starch and protein you are shoveling down; they will pass through your stomach untouched and leave you with a feeling of unpleasant heaviness.

If you drink while you are eating, you dilute your gastric juices, making them less effective, and this compounds the trouble. The food in your stomach ferments, producing bubbles of air, producing a feeling of bloat, and spasmodic belching.

At this point, many of us reach for a bicarbonate of soda, or some similar antacid preparation. This will produce relief, but if you carry it on too long you will find the cure becoming more uncomfortable than the disease. For your gastric glands will eventually get tired of all the extra work they are being subjected to, and instead of producing more acid they will produce less. The antacid you now take, instead of counteracting excess acid, will be neutralizing the little acid you have left and which you desperately need, so your stomach will virtually cease to act as a digestive organ. To get it going again you will need to eat something good and sour, like pickles in vinegar, before your meals.

It would be so much simpler to chew your food to begin with.

If you have got yourself into one of these gastric states, it may be necessary for you to go on a special diet for a short time to get your stomach back into normal working order.

First of all, make note of these general principles:

214

1) Try to eat as often as possible—four or five meals in the course of the day.

2) Rest a little before each meal.

3) Don't eat standing up. Sit down comfortably, take your time, don't get mad at anybody, and be sure to *chew*.

4) Don't drink during meals. Take your liquids in the half-hour preceding and following.

5) If you feel any discomfort during the course of the day, eat a piece of toast or drink a glass of milk.

6) Smoke only in the hour following meals. Or better still, don't smoke at all.

While you are giving your stomach a chance to quiet down, the following foods are strictly *forbidden*:

> All fatty meats
> All delicatessen products except lean ham
> Lard, or any cooked fat
> White or whole-wheat bread (toast, however, is all right)
> Whole-wheat cereals
> Dried vegetables
> The following fresh vegetables: cabbage, cauliflower, onion, garlic, spinach, radish, turnip, celery, cucumber
> All raw vegetables
> Oily fruits and nuts (olives, peanuts, etc.)
> Unripe fruits
> Rich desserts
> Fermented cheeses
> Soups made with meat, fish or any of the vegetables above
> In general, oversalted or oversugared foods
> Alcoholic beverages

You may or may not be able to support citrus fruits. Test them cautiously to see if your stomach approves.

With these out of the way, you can make up a daily ration something like this:

- *Breakfast:*
  A bowl of cereal with milk
  2 toasts with butter and jelly
  A very ripe fruit or a glass of fruit juice
  A small cup of light tea

- At *ten in the morning* (if possible):
  A yogurt or a glass of milk

- *Midday meal:*
  A cold vegetable, like beets, with oil and lemon juice
  A broiled, roasted or boiled piece of lean meat or fish
  A green vegetable or potatoes (or pasta or rice) boiled
    or steamed, with butter
  A mild cheese
  A very ripe fruit; or stewed fruit

- *Afternoon snack:*
  A glass of fruit juice or milk
  Dry crackers or biscuits

- *Evening meal:*
  A cooked vegetable with oil and lemon juice or a
    small portion of thick vegetable soup
  Meat or fish as above; or 2 eggs
  Potatoes or green vegetable (the one you didn't have
    for lunch)
  Cheese or light dessert

- At *ten at night:*
  A yogurt or a glass of milk or a milk-based dessert

A few weeks on this diet should calm your stomach down enough so that you can go back without difficulty to the standard Training Diet described in Chapter III.

INTESTINAL DISORDERS

There is an immense variety of these, and they are all the more insidious and dangerous because they can affect the organism in so many different ways that it is sometimes difficult to isolate the cause.

There are two major syndromes: ileo-colic stasis, better known as constipation, and colitis, or inflammation of the large intestine. Both of them, in addition to local discomfort, can cause migraine, vertigo, nausea, physical and mental fatigue, and fits of depression.

A common though often unsuspected cause of these symptoms is a parasitic infestation of the large intestine. This has nothing to do with your daily diet, but I mention it here because I have noticed it so often in athletes, particularly young men who have traveled abroad, and more particularly when they have traveled abroad in the armed services. I have known literally scores of such young men who have come down with unexpected and unexplained attacks of extreme fatigue and fits of intense anxiety and depression, a few years after they came home from army service in Indo-China or Algeria.

Their doctors were often all too eager to look for a psychiatric explanation, and they treated them for nervous breakdowns; in some cases they even hospitalized them. Again and again I found that what had happened was this: they had had a bout of dysentery overseas, but being young and vigorous they had come through it with no apparent after-effects. There were amoebas or other parasites still left in their colon, however, waiting to strike years later. If they had had malaria, the doctors would have had to recognize there was a physical cause, because of the high fever. But colitis brings no fever, and it is easy to misread its symptoms as signs of mental disturbance.

I am sure that many GI's who fought in Korea or Vietnam must have had the same experience.

Of course there are many other causes for intestinal troubles than parasites. They may be the result of an infection, or an allergy. Or they may be due to over indulgence in laxatives or to eating too much coarse cellulose, such as you may find in spinach, cabbage, and mushrooms.

You may need medical attention for your condition. But in any case, whatever the cause and whatever the symptoms—piles, diarrhea, or the more general ones described above—you will have to follow a diet that puts the least possible strain on your intestines.

The following foods are strictly *forbidden*:

Whole, powdered, or condensed milk
Fermented cheeses
Fat meats or fish
All delicatessen products except lean ham
Shellfish (except oysters)
Cooked fats and sauces
All raw vegetables
Cabbage, squash, cauliflower, spinach, turnip, cucumber, eggplant, green peas, radish, artichoke, mushrooms
All fresh fruits except apples, pears and peaches (all to be eaten quite ripe, and skinned) and citrus fruit juice
Dried fruits and nuts
White or whole wheat bread
Whole wheat cereal or oatmeal
Pastries, pancakes, chocolate, ice cream
Jam
Alcoholic beverages
Soda water

Here is a model day's menu:

• *Breakfast*:
  Cereal with skimmed milk

Light tea or coffee with sugar
Toast with butter and jelly (make sure it is jelly, not
    jam)
Juice of a citrus fruit

- *Midday meal:*
    Cooked vegetable with oil and vinegar
    Broiled, roasted or boiled meat or fish
    Potatoes or rice or pasta (alternating with a green
        vegetable)
    Mild cheese or yogurt
    Stewed fruit or ripe fresh fruit
    Toast

- *Afternoon snack*:
    Light tea with sugar
    A yogurt or a glass of skimmed milk
    Crackers or biscuits

- *Evening meal*:
    Strained vegetable soup with vermicelli or tapioca
    Meat or fish
    Green vegetable (alternating with potatoes or rice or
        pasta)
    A light dessert like a custard, with skimmed milk; or
        a yogurt
    Fruit juice

A note on occasional constipation:

It often happens that a system which is normally well regulated tightens up, perhaps as the result of a change in environment, on the day of the Event. If this seems to cause unnecessary discomfort, you may—on this occasion and on this occasion only—turn to a glycerin suppository to straighten you out.

LIVER AND GALL BLADDER DISORDERS

It is notorious that every Frenchman has liver trouble, and most of it is imaginary, though a source of very real profit to the owners of springs of mineral water and the like.

However, even a non-Frenchman must admit that the liver does exist, and though it is a very sturdy organ, things can and do go wrong with it.

Sometimes this is the result of infectious hepatitis which for a variety of reasons has become a scourge of the modern world. Infectious hepatitis is rarely fatal, but it can leave long-lasting and debilitating traces.

Or liver trouble can be the result of excessive consumption of food (especially fats) and alcohol, which put an undue strain on the liver cells.

Whatever its causes, liver trouble can be recognized by certain common symptoms: dry skin, thick tongue, sparse and strongly colored urine, discolored feces, etc.

And it takes a peculiar form which I have often observed in athletes: it attacks the muscles and tendons. I believe I was the first to point out this phenomenon, in the case of a French broad-jumping champion named Christian Collardot who was continually getting in trouble because he was always getting his muscles pulled or torn when he went into training. I discovered that he had once had a bout of infectious hepatitis, and after he was treated for that he had no more problems and went on to win several championships. The connection between liver trouble and muscles and tendon weakness is now well established.

Accidents will happen on the training and playing field. But if they happen suspiciously often in this form, it is a good idea to have your liver tested.

If there is something wrong with it, this is what you can do about it, nutritionally speaking.

The following foods are *forbidden*:

All forms of fat meat
Salted, smoked, canned or fatty fish
Shellfish
All forms of animal fat
Gravies and sauces
Cabbage, cauliflower, squash, spinach, turnip, cucumber, celery, onion, garlic
Spices
Oily fruits and nuts
Pastry, desserts, candy
Alcoholic drinks
Soda water
Iced drinks

The following foods should be taken only in strictly limited quantities:

Butter: 10 grams a day (or 20 of cream)
Oil: 20 grams a day (or 30 of margarine)
2 eggs a week, but only if your system can take them
Fermented cheese, 2 or 3 times a week, but again, only if your system can take it

You can take what you want of the following foods, but first make sure you have no reaction to them:

Whole milk (if you can't take whole milk replace it by skimmed milk or yogurt, and in this case increase your butter ration to 20 grams)
Carrots, artichokes, leeks, tomatoes, green peas
Dried vegetables
Strawberries, raspberries, plums, pineapple, bananas

Here is a model daily ration:

• *Breakfast*:
A bowl of cereal with whole or skimmed milk

A cup of tea or coffee with sugar
Toast and jelly or jam
Fruit or fresh fruit juice

- *Midday meal*:
  1 raw or cooked vegetable with oil and lemon juice
  Broiled, roasted or boiled meat or fish
  1 green vegetable or 1 starchy product (potatoes, pasta, rice) boiled or steamed, with melted butter
  1 piece of cheese or yogurt
  1 ripe fruit, or stewed fruit

- *Afternoon snack*:
  1 yogurt or 1 glass of whole or skimmed milk
  Crackers or biscuits

- *Evening meal*:
  Strained vegetable soup with vermicelli or tapioca
  Meat or fish, as above (no gravy of course)
  Starch or green vegetable (whichever you didn't have for lunch)
  Cheese
  1 ripe fruit, or stewed fruit

DENTAL CAVITIES

In the modern world, dental decay is almost always caused by defective diet. Athletes in particular should pay attention to this, because at moments of intense nervous pressure the forces of pain are apt to settle in on any weakness your body may present. If the weakness is in your teeth, you will regret it. The moment of the Event for which you have been preparing for weeks is hardly the time you would choose for a toothache, with grotesquely swollen cheek and excruciating stabs of pain going up into the very center of your brain.

The main cause of tooth decay is overnourishment, particularly in refined sugar. This was illustrated dramatically enough in Europe in World War II, when there was a terrible prevalence of deficiency diseases but peoples' teeth were in better shape than normal. The reason was that no sugar could be imported into Europe during those years.

Sugar hurts your teeth in two ways. It predisposes your mouth for the breeding of the micrococcus *acidophilus*. And, especially if you eat it in the form of candy between meals, some of it gets stuck between your teeth and begins to ferment there, forming a little pocket of possible infection.

To protect your teeth, keep your ingestion of sugar down within the limits I have indicated: never more than 10% of your daily caloric intake. And make sure that you are not short of vitamins B and C. These rules go double for adolescents, for at their stage of growth the teeth are particularly vulnerable.

A helpful hint I have mentioned earlier is to eat an apple at bedtime. The pectin in the apple will dissolve sugar lodged between your teeth.

MINOR RESPIRATORY INFECTIONS

I am afraid I cannot offer you a cure for the common cold. But I have noticed again and again that athletes who come down regularly with rhino-pharyngitis, sore throats and bronchial infections every time the weather turns bad are just the ones who have not been eating enough fruits and green vegetables regularly and who are therefore short of necessary vitamins, especially vitamin C. A little change in diet can often do wonders for these pesky diseases. A three-year study on 1,300 student volunteers at the University of Michigan is said to have shown that those who ate one apple a day had one-third fewer respiratory infections than those who neglected this simple form of alimentary prophylaxis. (They also had less trouble with their nerves.) These results seem to me to be somewhat on the miraculous side, but there is no doubt that an apple a day will do you good. Three apples might do more.

BOILS

Boils may be a reaction of the organism to local irritants, like tight-fitting clothing which rubs the skin and prevents the evaporation of sweat. Or sometimes there are more deep-seated causes: physical effort can set up a vitaminic disequilibrium and hypersecretion of the adrenal glands which render the body more liable to inflammation and then to infection. Eating too much refined sugar (often as the result of being in a pre-diabetic state) and going short of vitamins B and C can be contributing factors as well.

If you have boils, the first thing is to remove any cause of local irritation and keep the area clean. Then cut down on your carbohydrate intake by reducing your sugar consumption to half. Make sure that animal proteins make up no more than half of your daily protein ration. Take a few Vitamin B and C pills. And above all, try to improve your state of mind, for there is a strong psychosomatic factor in most outbreaks of boils.

PRE-MENSTRUAL DIFFICULTIES

These, of course, do not constitute a disease; they are part of the normal cycle of life. But it is common for women athletes to be disturbed at the approach of their periods, and they are naturally anxious to make sure that this does not interfere with their performance.

All too often efforts have been proposed, and actually made, to interfere chemically and postpone or suppress the ovulation which causes the menstrual flow. This is playing a dangerous game with a young woman's future health for the sake of a momentary satisfaction, and I heartily disapprove of all such experiments.

Nevertheless, I agree that it is desirable to do something to alleviate the nervous tension, and the feeling of heaviness in abdomen and breasts that is often experienced at this time. Some changes in the daily diet can help in these respects:

1) Cut down on your intake of salt. The feeling of heaviness comes from water piling up in your body, and we have already seen that salt helps retain water in your tissues. Ordinarily you want to do that at a time of physical effort, but this is one occasion when you will be glad to get rid of it.

2) But despite what you might think after reading the above paragraph, this is a time to drink *more* water than usual. It won't hang around and clog up your system. Water is the best diuretic known, and the more you drink, the less your tissues will retain.

3) Increase your consumption of vitamins A and B_1.

4) Eat more proteins, the same amount of carbohydrates, and less fats than usual. The blood has a higher fat content at this part of the menstrual process, so you can afford to cut down on your intake of fats.

5) And on the whole, eat a little more than usual.

OLD AGE

This is not a disease either, but no one can deny that it has its discomforts.

Sooner or later we all have to give up the active sports which our bodies could handle with no trouble in the days of our youth. This should be a gradual slacking off of activity, but all too often it is abrupt, and accompanied by a general loss of interest in the state of the general health of the body. We sit when we should be standing, ride when we should be walking, watch television reports of activities that we should be taking part in ourselves. Along with this, the principles of rational nutrition are apt to go overboard, partly because we can now afford to pay for indulgences which were impossible when we were trying to scrape together the down payment on the mortgage.

The consequences can be read in the statistics of increased diabetes, heart disease and God knows how many other disorders, in increased aches and pains and disgruntlement, in increased hospital bills.

There is little reason for all this except sheer laziness. It is hard to say that anyone these days lacks the time or opportunity to indulge in a small amount of body-maintaining exercise every day or at least a few times a week. On every side we see people, many of them aged or aging, who do find the time and opportunity and we can see them all over the place, biking, jogging, playing golf.

These are all worthy activities and I recommend them highly to the senior citizen—as long as he doesn't insist on following, say, the golf game with an interminable session at the 19th hole, recounting his exploits as the drinks pile up, and then go off to a seven-course dinner.

The nutritional rules laid down in this book, the standard ration spelled out in Chapter III, the remarks on the various foods in Chapter IV, the suggestions and hints scattered through the text, are all just as applicable when you are old as when you are in the full bloom of youth. You will naturally eat somewhat less as you grow older, at least if you listen to your body and not to your sometimes perverse tastes. You are less active and need fewer reserves of energy. Your basal metabolism diminishes as you age and you need fewer calories to keep it going. Your very frame is smaller—your vertebrae squeeze closer together over the years, your feet flatten—so you get shorter, and the shorter you are the less you weigh, or should weigh. For all these reasons you will be eating somewhat less food. (You will, however, be drinking more water because your body tends to dry out the closer it gets to the end of its course.)

But the food should be in the same proportions it was before and hopefully it will keep you in the same state of good health and good spirits.

Before I end, I would like to make a modest profession of faith in nutrition and what it can do for the future well-being of mankind.

I would not like to put myself among the army of enthusiasts and quacks who burst periodically on the scene to announce that a single product or combination of products (perhaps one in which, more or less coincidentally, they have a financial interest) is going to cure all the ills that man is heir to, wipe out cancer and the common cold, turn old age into springtime bliss, etc. The real world is not that simple.

It is in fact very complicated, and we progress in learning about it only by slow and tentative steps. I am convinced that all the impressive progress we have made so far is only a beginning, and that there are many factors still unknown or half-suspected which will one day help reshape our lives in the direction of better health, better use of all the resources of the human mind and body.

I think we have much to learn from the ecological movement which is making so much of a commotion these days. It is perhaps overequipped with zealots who are prone to exaggeration and sometimes plain nonsense, and we have to guard against the nonsense.

I am not, for example, prepared to follow the enthusiasts who would give up all the fruits of thousands of years of painful progress toward civilization for the sake of going back to a natural paradise which I suspect never existed except in the imagination of the ecologists themselves.

They are right in saying that we eat a much narrower

range of food than our prehistoric ancestors. Those ancestors knew and used more than 2,000 kinds of plant life, while it is rare that we taste more than a couple of dozen in the course of a year. The plants we eat are the ones that can be conveniently grown by modern agricultural methods. Primitive man had a richer choice.

Let us not romanticize those faroff ancestors for all that. Most of those 2,000 plants would be found frankly uneatable by our finicky modern tastes, and some of them—like the bark of birch trees—are considered unfit for the human stomach by modern nutritionists. (It is true that they may have been used for medicinal purposes we can only guess at.) The forebears of our tender modern green peas were coarse fibrous beans which probably tore up the intestines of Primitive Man more than they nourished him.

Nor was Primitive Man quite the paragon of good health that modern primitivists like to imagine. He had arthritis, he had bad teeth, and generally he died quite young.

We are in fact healthier today than at any other time in the previous history of mankind. There may have been in the past isolated individuals or tribes who found themselves in exceptional environments and lived on a superior level of health. But the general level has always been pretty low, by today's standards. Living close to the soil has not made necessarily for good diet or good health. There was no one around in prehistoric times to perform autopsies, but we do have records of autopsies in the Middle Ages, beginning with Maimonides and other Jewish physicians at the courts of Moslem Spain. The scale and profusion of parasitic life that flourished inside the human body in those days, as revealed by such records, is absolutely appalling to modern eyes; we find it hard to believe that people could have lived, let alone functioned, under such conditions. Modern hygiene and, yes, modern insecticides have really helped our health considerably by getting rid of enormous quantities of filth of all sorts that made life a much more chancy business then than it is today.

Having said all this, I will say that I think the ecologists are on the right track when they say that we have unnecessarily narrowed our range of dietary interest. Instead of looking for the foods that are best for us, we have looked for the ones that are, technologically speaking, the easiest to produce.

It is only natural for research funds to be directed toward the development of improved strains of tomato rather than the discovery and testing of obscure jungle plants. But the latter may have their riches to offer us, as was proved spectacularly not long ago when rawulfia, product of a faroff Pacific island, was found to make an invaluable contribution to the treatment of both arterial diseases and mental depression.

I am sure that there are many more such discoveries to be made, not just medicinal in nature but broadening the range of foods that keep us in good health.

In Tollund in Denmark not so long ago they dug up a body about 2,000 years old, that of a man who had been thrown into a peat-bog, naked except for a cap on his head and a noose around his neck. It is assumed that he was hanged as part of a religious ceremony and buried as an offering to the earth gods or goddesses who cause food to sprout out of the soil.

The body of the Tollund man was perfectly preserved, including his stomach, which still retained his last, undigested meal. This meal consisted of no less than 144 plants, berries, and herbs of all descriptions.

Some of these are considered poisonous today, but for all we know others may have been antidotes. In fact, we know very little about most of these herbs, except perhaps their Latin names. I like to think that someday an analysis of all the food in the stomach of that unfortunate ancient Dane may open the way to new discoveries that will widen our knowledge of nutrition and perhaps significantly improve our lives. I look for much more genuine progress in this way than in the creation of synthetic artificial stimulants to help a runner or swimmer gain a couple of tenths of a second in some race.

We live in a technological, largely synthetic world, but the bodies we were born with still have their own knowledge, and I believe we will do best in the long run by trusting them. That, I hope, is the message of this book.

231

234

238

241

242

245

HORROR BESTSELLERS
by J.N. Williamson
FOR THOSE COLD, LONELY NIGHTS!

DEATH-COACH (805, $2.95)
A young woman and her children become the innocent victims of horrifying evil when they move into a small quiet town inhabited by the bloodthirsty Queen of Vampires, Lamia Zacharius.

DEATH-ANGEL (909, $2.95)
Disguised as a beautiful woman, Lamia Zacharius, the three-thousand-year-old vampire, creates the most monstrous child the world has ever known.

DEATH-SCHOOL (981, $2.95)
Thessaly's lovely new school teacher is the deadly vampire Lamia Zacharius—and the children are headed for a horrifying course of evil from which there is no return!

DEATH-DOCTOR (1108, $2.95)
As the lovely "doctor" Lamia Zacharius, Queen of the Vampires, cradles a scarlet-eyed infant in her arms she croons with hideous delight. For this newborn is the essence of all that is evil: a deadly, horrifying demon who hungers for fresh human blood . . .

Available wherever paperbacks are sold, or order direct from the Publisher. Send cover price plus 50¢ per copy for mailing and handling to Zebra Books, 475 Park Avenue South, New York, N.Y. 10016. DO NOT SEND CASH.

THE SURVIVALIST SERIES
by Jerry Ahern

#1: TOTAL WAR   (960, $2.50)
The first in the shocking series that follows the unrelenting search for ex-CIA covert operations officer John Thomas Rourke to locate his missing family—after the button is pressed, the missiles launched and the multimegaton bombs unleashed . . .

#2: THE NIGHTMARE BEGINS   (810, $2.50)
After WW III, the United States is just a memory. But ex-CIA covert operations officer Rourke hasn't forgotten his family. While hiding from the Soviet occupation forces, he adheres to his search!

#3: THE QUEST   (851, $2.50)
Not even a deadly game of intrigue within the Soviet High Command, the formation of the American "resistance" and a highly placed traitor in the new U.S. government can deter Rourke from continuing his desperate search for his family.

#4: THE DOOMSAYER   (893, $2.50)
The most massive earthquake in history is only hours away, and Communist-Cuban troops, Soviet-Cuban rivalry, and a traitor in the inner circle of U.S. II block Rourke's path. But he must go on—he is THE SURVIVALIST.

#5: THE WEB   (1145, $2.50)
Blizzards rage around Rourke as he picks up the trail of his family and is forced to take shelter in a strangely quiet Tennessee valley town. Things seem too normal here, as if no one has heard of the War; but the quiet isn't going to last for long!

Available wherever paperbacks are sold, or order direct from the Publisher. Send cover price plus 50¢ per copy for mailing and handling to Zebra Books, 475 Park Avenue South, New York, N.Y. 10016. DO NOT SEND CASH.